Understanding Low Back Pain

Understanding Low Back Pain

Breakthroughs and New Advances in the Diagnosis and Treatment of Low Back Pain

New Concept: Evidence-Based Medicine applied in the Treatment of LBP

MARIO A. GUTIERREZ, MD

iUniverse, Inc.

New York Lincoln Shanghai

Understanding Low Back Pain
Breakthroughs and New Advances in the Diagnosis and Treatment of Low
Back Pain

iUniverse books may be ordered through booksellers or by contacting:

iUniverse
2021 Pine Lake Road, Suite 100
Lincoln, NE 68512
www.iuniverse.com
1-800-Authors (1-800-288-4677)

I obtained permission for the use of statistical, disability and medical
information from the:

• American Medical Association
• New England Journal of Medicine

Some information contained in this book can be obtained in most medical
textbooks, Internet, medical journals and other publications. Accurate statistical
information and medical references are available also at the same sources.

I created the drawings contained in this book. I made also some quotations
throughout this book. I described some new medical entities not published
yet in medical textbooks, but this information may stimulate research centers
for further scientific investigation.

ISBN-13: 978-0-595-34117-7 (pbk)
ISBN-13: 978-0-595-67065-9 (cloth)
ISBN-13: 978-0-595-78894-1 (ebk)
ISBN-10: 0-595-34117-9 (pbk)
ISBN-10: 0-595-67065-2 (cloth)
ISBN-10: 0-595-78894-7 (ebk)

Printed in the United States of America

CONTENTS

ACKNOWLEDGMENTS

It took me over three years to complete this book. I did not know how hard it is to put together so many thoughts in an organized way. I did not realize how much support is needed from different people in the making of a book.

For that reason, I thank very much the people that helped me complete this book. I also want to dedicate this book to people that have meant a great deal to me. I especially thank my mother, who, as a single mother, saw me through my studies and encouraged me to continue the arduous road of medical school and residency.

I thank my wife, Ilsa, for supporting me emotionally through my fellowships and for sharing with me the very difficult years of my fellowships in San Antonio, Texas, and Baltimore, Maryland, and for her continuing support during the last seventeen years.

I thank my children, Alex and Vanessa, for their support and encouragement. Alex, my twelve-year-old son, helped me with some ideas with the use of the computer and camera equipment and with some of the drawings in this book.

I dedicate this book especially:

To the thousands of patients I have had the privilege of treating and for allowing me to be their physician. Thanks to them, I was able to write this book. I dedicate this book to them as a token of my gratitude because their pain and suffering will help others.

To my deceased brother, Rodolfo, and surviving brother, Alfredo, and my sister, Laura.

To my dear friend, Dr. Ramesh Nayak, who recently passed away and left a great legacy of ethics and knowledge to me.

To my dear friend, Maurice Musik, who taught me the value of courage.

To Linda Gonzalez and Emma Arzola, who helped by proofreading my original manuscript.

To all my close friends.

DISCLAIMER

This book is by no means intended to be a substitute for your physician's advice. It does not intend to cover all aspects of the lower back, the spine, or medicine in general.

Some of the information included in this book is a compilation of personal medical experience and objective basic medical information contained in most textbooks, journals, and magazines related to disorders of the lower back. This book contains general concepts not obtained from one specific book, journal, or magazine. Basic concepts and statistical information can be further found in any research paper, medical journal, or library.

I recommend readers use this book only as an educational and informative source. It may be used to assist patients with LBP in making more reasonable inquiries to their physician. Education and knowledge are invaluable tools. One does not know what to ask if there is a lack of essential knowledge.

This book does not intend to debase any particular institution or physician, nor does it intend to make rules out of my concepts. Some of my concepts and recommendations may apply to some people, but not to others.

This is not an official medical textbook. It contains information related to the spine and particularly the lower back. The intention of this book is to help individuals understand conditions that affect the lower back in a more rational and clear way.

It is not my intention to promote any specific treatment, medical company, surgical device, or equipment. I strongly recommend a person with LBP seek professional medical advice regarding any of the issues covered in this book. I recognize that some of the subjects of this book can be subject to controversy and debate.

The information contained in this book may not be updated. The author is not responsible for injury or loss due to the application of information contained in this book. The author does not accept responsibility for the accuracy validity and reliability of this book. This is not a legal document and may not uphold in a court of law. I do not recommend using this book for legal matters in arbitration and for legal actions. This is not an authoritative book.

I recommend consulting appropriate sources of information from medical textbooks and national statistics and checking other resources for a more complete definition of some terms used in this book.

INTRODUCTION

I decided to write this book about the lower back because I have seen many patients with low back pain (LBP) who had unanswered questions. I noticed confusion among insurance companies, patients, and even some physicians concerning the diagnosis and treatment of patients with LBP. I felt it was important to write a book designed for the layman but that would also benefit medical students, athletes, or anyone who has an interest in knowing more about the human body. However, I primarily wanted to assist the public in avoiding injuries of the spine (particularly the lower back) because these injuries may be carried for a lifetime.

This book is not only designed for the person with LBP; it also contains information for the general public. I think that, by reading this book, people will prevent back injuries. Prevention is the key to decrease the incidence of sickness. I expect with this book to save the system (that is, economy) hundreds—possibly millions—of dollars by teaching the public the causes and most frequent treatments of this condition that affect so many people in the world. I also want to inform the public of the nuances in the diagnosis and treatment of the patient with LBP.

Physicians in private practice often make clinical observations and discoveries through years of experience that, for several reasons, are never published in any medical publication. Physicians like me, who are in private practice, do not have the time or the means to publish these observations. We only share the observations with other colleagues and refer to them as "pearls." Frequently, there is professional jealousy, and these observations are not shared in the medical community.

These unpublished clinical observations are a very important part of the "everyday medical practice," and they are considered to be components of what is known as Evidence-Based Medicine (EBM).

EBM is the practice of medicine based on the expertise of the physician. Expertise in a field or profession is gained over time, and it is based on basic training, solid known scientific information, experience, and intuition all used for the benefit of the patient. By combining these factors, EBM offers the best possible treatment for a particular patient.

EBM provides treatment for the patient with a specific medical condition. It is not only used in writing publications; it is used for the decision-making process. However, it acknowledges scientifically collected data. Physicians and other professionals tend to think in a linear cause-effect manner. We expect to have a particular solution for a particular problem. Medicine is not an equation as some physicians try to make it. There are no perfect guidelines, flowcharts, and algorithms that will give us an answer when we speak of the diagnosis and treatment of the patient with LBP.

The application of EBM is not easy to define. A thin line separates medical objective data from intangible information. Some call it intuition, hunches, and so forth. EBM is an approach from different angles and perspectives in order to treat a patient. No computer program will give us the exact answer to treat a patient with certain medical conditions. We are still trying to understand the functions of the different organs and systems in the human body. There are several treatment options for certain problems in medicine.

We physicians attempt to master the difficult area of EBM throughout our careers, but our efforts require a great deal of practice, reading, learning, experience, common sense, reasoning, and intuition. If there is an equation in medicine, it would probably be the following: Objective Evidence [Medical Data] + Subjective Evidence [Symptoms] + Medical Interpretation [Experience] + Common Sense = Outcome. Albert Einstein once said, "I went into physics and mathematics because I do not like inexact and unpredictable sciences such as medicine."

I have seen hundreds of patients while practicing neurosurgery for more than twenty years. Most of these patients usually asked the same questions, and many of them had misconceptions relating to the lower back. There is still a great deal of misunderstanding when we refer to the diagnosis and treatment of the person with LBP.

It is common that people misinterpret isolated information obtained from sources such as books, the Internet, medical boards, spine institutes, clinics, and magazines with special articles about LBP. It is completely understandable that patients with LBP would want to know all about the lower back, but the information they accumulate sometimes only serves to confuse them. One should not take one single source of information as the only truth. People tend to make a consistent rule out of one source of information. Not all patients with LBP are the same; not all back conditions have a common cause. I may repeat this statement throughout the book only to emphasize the importance of treating patients with LBP individually.

With this book, I want to share the observations and implementations I have designed during my years of practice. I want to share the benefits of alternative medicine with those who are eager to learn about their anatomy and who care about their health and with those who have an open mind for alternative healing techniques. When I wrote this book, I felt compelled to share my experience in using EBM so that the public would develop a better understanding of the lower back.

In order to cover all aspects of the lower back, I would need to write volumes of information; however, some facts, which are "pearls," will be presented in this book. This book summarizes information contained in textbooks, journals, magazines, and so forth, but, more importantly, it conveys several years of my personal experiences, my opinions, and my suggestions, all compiled and explained in lay terms. This reading can be considered typical EBM (that is, concepts and opinions). It is primarily intended for the general public, but it is also for those interested in starting a medical career, for practicing physicians, nurses and other. At the end of each chapter, there is a section of questions. I think the reader will find substantial information.

There is medical terminology and a short medical glossary at the end of this book. Also, at the end of this book, there is a section with some of the most frequent medical abbreviations. I have included my own drawings—that may not be highly artistic—but they are designed only to convey an idea. I suggest referring to the anatomy and glossary sections when reading this book.

When I read a book, I sometimes feel tempted to skip some sections to get to the part that interests me the most, but, commonly, one has to follow a chronological order or to follow chapter after chapter to understand the entire book. When I wrote this book, I divided it into sections that can be read independently without the need to follow one order. If the reader is interested in the treatment of patients with LBP, surgery, frequency of LBP, anatomy of the spine, and so forth, the reader can refer to a specific section. However, I recommend reading the entire book to understand all aspects of the patient with LBP.

Instead of making only a technical book about patients with LBP, causes, frequency, treatment, and so forth, I decided to include aspects of the patient with LBP, that, in a sense, have some influence in the global understanding of these patients: insurance information, pitfalls in radiological interpretation and in treatment, personal comments, and, mostly, aspects related to EBM.

I will use the abbreviation LBP when referring to LBP throughout this book. I may seem to be redundant with some concepts in some sections of this book, but I want to emphasize certain points I consider important. Each chapter has a section of questions and answers, and I sometimes refer to the same issues in the questions that have already been addressed in the preceding chapter. At the end of each chapter, I have included drawings to depict the anatomy of the spine, radiological pictures, various spinal conditions, and surgical techniques.

"Medicine is a science and an art, and the ability to combine them with psychomotor skills, knowledge, compassion, and honesty is what makes the greatest healers. Those who lack any of these qualities may place patients at risk."
M.A. Gutierrez, MD

After reading this book, the reader will learn:

- The frequency of LBP in the population and its economical impact on our society
- Basic anatomy and biomechanics of the spine
- Different medical specialties related to the treatment of LBP
- Causes of LBP
- Most frequent studies used for the diagnosis of LBP
- Treatment options
- History of back surgery
- What to expect before and after surgery
- Indications and contraindications of surgery
- Different surgical techniques
- Complications of the different treatments
- Rehabilitation/Prevention of LBP injuries
- Myths in the treatment of patients with LBP
- Updated treatment of patients with LBP (artificial disc implant or disc replacement)
- Personal concepts in the treatment of patients with LBP
- The functions of a medical office and insurance companies (workers' compensation); disability evaluation
- Example of management in typical cases of LBP
- Future treatment (gene therapy)
- Medical abbreviations and glossary

CHAPTER 1

Basic Information

How Frequent is LBP? Epidemiological information

There are costs involved not only for the treatment of someone with low back pain (LBP), but also for other socioeconomic issues related to the patient with LBP such as litigation, work time missed, replaced personnel, retraining, vocational rehabilitation, disability, compensations, fraud and so forth. It is a domino effect affecting the patient and the family, and it has social and economic implications.

Some patients with LBP lose their jobs and apply for Social Security or disability; some are classified as nontaxable, working people. Some people qualify for Medicaid; others qualify for different government benefits: all of which the taxpayers fund.

In many aspects, LBP is a major problem in our society. There are studies that analyze the costs incurred in the treatment of patients with LBP. Some of these studies do not include several of the factors mentioned above; therefore, they may not be entirely accurate in calculating the actual figure.

It has been calculated that the prevalence and lifetime incidence of LBP can be as high as eighty-five to ninety percent, which means that up to ninety percent of the population between the ages of eighteen and sixty-five will experience LBP at some point in their lives. There is no clear difference between the male and female population in the incidence of LBP. While some studies suggest it is more prevalent in females, other studies point to males. These percentages may vary by country and by the particular socioeconomic structure of the population. About one-third of the population over the age of forty-five has chronic LBP. LBP is the leading cause of disability in people under forty.

In the United States, it has been calculated that over 4.5 million people are disabled due to LBP or related conditions. Between ten and twenty percent of adults have LBP, resulting in thirteen million physician visits per year. LBP is one of the most frequently diagnosed conditions resulting in ten percent of all chronic medical diagnoses. It is estimated that, in the United States, there are about six to seven million cases of LBP every year. Twenty-two percent of all work-related accidents are back injuries.

LBP is also the most frequent cause of physical limitations being placed on people under sixty-four, and it is the most frequent cause of missed work by individuals between the ages of twenty-five and forty-four. An average of thirty days per one hundred workers is lost each year due to LBP, and it is the fifth-ranking cause of hospitalization. LBP is also the second-ranking reason for visits to the physician after heart conditions. In addition, low back conditions are the third-ranking reason for surgical intervention and the most frequent and expensive cause of work-related disability in people under forty-five.

Family practitioners, chiropractors, osteopathic doctors, neurosurgeons, orthopedic surgeons, physiatrists (that is, specialists in physical medicine and rehabilitation), occupational medicine specialists, neurologists, and physiotherapists typically treat patients suffering from LBP.

It is estimated that about fifty billion dollars are spent annually in direct health care costs in the U.S. for the care of patients with LBP. However, if you include indirect costs associated with LBP, it has been estimated that as much as ninety billion dollars, with an average of twenty-six billion dollars, are spent in the United States for LBP and related issues. Twenty billion dollars are spent on LBP claims in work-related injuries.

Even though there is a high prevalence of LBP in this country and the economic impact upon our government, insurance companies, and the taxpayers is great, there is still no common consensus relating to the treatment of a patient with acute and chronic LBP.

I sincerely believe this book will help people understand lower back conditions. I also think that, by reading this book, people (that is, patients, insurance companies, and physicians) could help the global economy, particularly the health system. The economy of our country may save millions—or billions—of dollars with the information contained in this book. These savings could specifically be accomplished by considering the information relating to the prevention of low back injuries and by choosing more reasonable treatment plans presented here. I suggest consulting reputable scientific information for confirmation of statistical data.

Anatomy of the Lumbar Spine

The spine is a complex piece of biological engineering. It is an anthropological and biological adaptation to our nature and environment. The mechanics and the structure of the spine are integral factors that contribute to our survival and our everyday functions. However, due to our erect position and our continual aging process, the spine also ages, as does any other organ in our body. The spine, in particular, can cause several painful conditions as it ages and suffers mechanical changes.

The spine is divided in regions or zones:

From the top down, it is the cervical (neck), thoracic (upper back), and lumbar spine (lower back). The lower part of the spine is called the sacrum bone, and the very tip of the spine or tailbone is the coccyx. Seven bones, or vertebrae, are in the cervical spine, twelve bones are in the thoracic spine, and five bones are in the lumbar spine. The sacrum bone is one single piece (that is, a rudimentary fusion of five vertebrae). The coccyx is also one single piece that consists of fused, rudimentary vertebrae. We refer to the vertebrae as "C" for cervical, "T" or "D" for thoracic or dorsal, "L" for lumbar, and "S" for sacrum. An L4-5 disc would be the disc between the fourth and the fifth lumbar vertebra. The L5-S1 disc is the one between the fifth lumbar vertebra and the sacrum.

The spinal cord and the nerves are inside the spine. The nerves exit the spinal canal through holes called foramen. A sheath or membrane called dura cover the spinal cord and the nerves, just like a coating covers electrical wires. Inside the dura and surrounding the spinal cord is spinal fluid. The vertebral column normally has certain curvatures in the cervical, thoracic, lumbar spine, and in the sacrum and coccyx. Exaggeration of the normal curves of the spine may lead to painful conditions and deformity of the spine (for example, lordosis, kyphosis, rotoscoliosis, and scoliosis).

The vertebrae lay one on top of the other and over the joints, discs, and vertebral bodies. There are ligaments, tendons, and muscles holding this complex structure.

The flat surface of the vertebral bodies is made of cartilage called "end plates" that cover and protect the surfaces of the vertebral bodies. Around this structure is a ligament called annulus fibrosis. Inside this ligament in the center of the space between the vertebral bodies in the flat surface is the nucleus pulposus is a gelatin-like substance that occupies only one-third of the center of the intervertebral space. Surrounding ligaments hold the disc in place. Ruptures or tears of these ligaments with escape of the inner gelatin-like nucleus pulposus substance is known as a protruding disc. The protruding portion of the disc pinches a nerve root and causes LBP and/or leg pain. Other symptoms may accompany a disc herniation. I will mention these situations later in this book. Several terms are used for these events: slipped disc, ruptured disc, herniated disc or disc herniation, extruded disc, bulging disc, and so forth. I will mention these conditions later in this book.

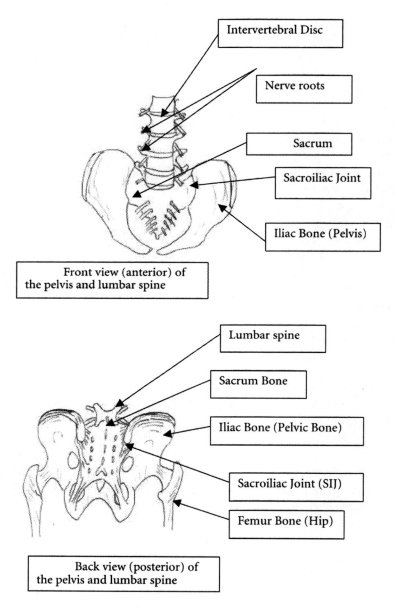

Front view (anterior) of
the pelvis and lumbar spine

Back view (posterior) of
the pelvis and lumbar spine

LBP can be caused by different disorders in the lower back affecting one or more structures such as muscles, ligaments, tendons, joints, and bones. The sacroiliac joint is one of the most frequent sources of pain, and it tends to be confused with spinal conditions.

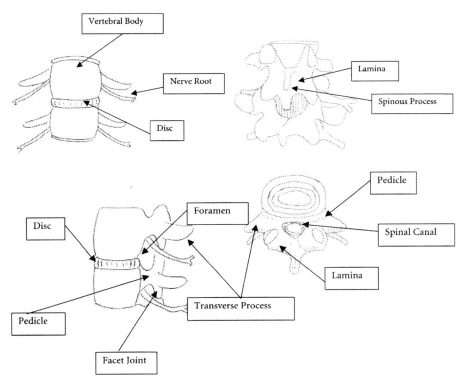

From upper to lower and from left to right: Front View (Anterior), Back View (Posterior), Side View (Lateral) and Up-down View (Axial) of a vertebra.

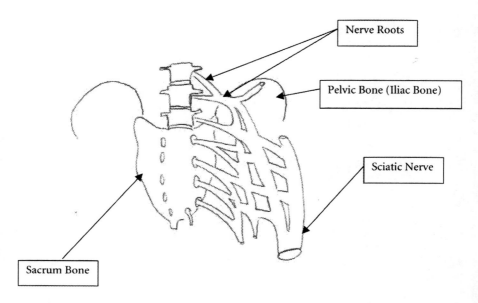

Nerve Roots

Pelvic Bone (Iliac Bone)

Sciatic Nerve

Sacrum Bone

Front view of the pelvis. After the nerve roots exit the spinal canal through the foramen (holes in the vertebrae), they fuse (or merge) together and make larger nerves such as the sciatic nerve made of the nerve roots L4, L5, S1, S2, and S3. Anything affecting any of these nerve roots can cause "sciatic" pain. The sciatic nerve can also be pinched as it travels behind the hip and down anywhere in the leg. Cluster of nerves make what is called plexus.

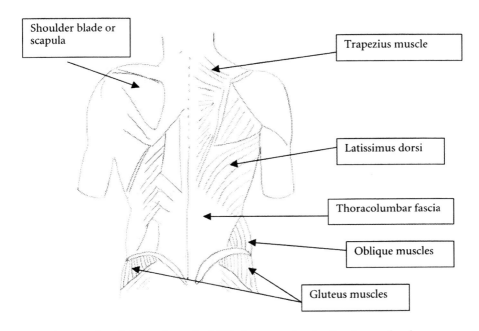

Shoulder blade or scapula

Trapezius muscle

Latissimus dorsi

Thoracolumbar fascia

Oblique muscles

Gluteus muscles

Back muscles. When there is LBP, the muscles in the lower back are con-nected to other muscles all the way to the upper back and up to the neck. Therefore, LBP can be associated with a chronic strain affecting not only the lower back but also the upper back and the neck. Patients commonly complain of pain "all over." Patients tend to complain of headaches as well. After back surgery, the muscles may lose some fibers. This can lead to atrophy of the mus-cles and chronic LBP. Some low back exercises are indicated after surgery to keep the muscles strong. However, one must be cautious on the timing for back exercises. Strenuous exercises performed early after surgery may cause more LBP and muscle spasms. Muscles, tendons, and ligaments are important structures to maintain the alignment of the spine. They are the main support-ing structures of the spine. Muscle-related conditions such as chronic strain are the leading cause of LBP in general.

Biomechanics of the Lower Back

Physics and mechanics are directly associated with our complex anatomical structure known as the spine. In fact, it is gravity and the curvature of the spine that support the human body in an erect manner. It has been assumed that the erect position of humans leads to spinal deterioration. Indeed, this may be a contributing factor. The spine gives us the ability to stand upright and to walk. Unfortunately, it is still my opinion the spine is doomed to deteriorate at the lowest point, possibly due to gravity effect. Areas of the spine that are under physical stress tend to deteriorate early in life. There are four-legged animals that also experience spinal deterioration and defy the gravity theory of spinal deterioration (due to the upright posture). Spinal deterioration relentlessly occurs as we age.

The spine, or backbone, is expected to deteriorate as we age. Other factors such as genetic influence (hereditary conditions), poor posture, physical activities (sports), obesity, smoking, diabetes, and other mechanical and medical conditions determine when someone will have spinal problems. We tend to believe that what makes us stand straight is the strength of the spine, but the spine itself would be able to carry only a few pounds if it were left without all the ligaments, muscles, and tendons, the real supporting structures. This is the reason why LBP is usually related to strained muscles rather than true to spinal (bones or discs) conditions. Aging and prolonged or extended strain on the muscles can cause degenerative spine changes that ultimately lead to spur formation, spinal stenosis, and slipped discs. Other factors can also accelerate the aging or degenerative process. I will discuss more about causes of LBP in the next chapters of this book.

LBP is not a matter of *if* it is going to happen but *when* it is going to happen. Refer to the epidemiological chapter for more details. There are ways to delay or avoid early deterioration of the spine. Although it has not been proven scientifically, there are contradictory reports on the cause or aggravation of spinal conditions when referring to physical activities and posture.

Researchers have developed a method of measuring the pressure inside the disc in different situations and positions. This measurement is called intradiscal pressure, or IDP. IDP has been measured after applying different loads to the spine and after bending. IDP has been measured during different physical activities and positions of the spine. IDP is measured in newtons.

The intradiscal pressure increases double and triple fold at thirty-five pounds and over. For instance, when lying down, the intradiscal pressure may be 400 newtons. (This is not necessarily an accurate example in physics, but it is sufficient to convey the idea.) Standing, the IDP may increase to 800 or 1000 newtons. The action of lifting over thirty-five pounds increases the IDP directly proportional to the load and inversely to the resistance of the soft tissues and disc resistance, and it will definitely increase the IDP well over 1000 newtons.

The action of bending is a force that increases IDP; the force associated with shear loading and bending of the spine. (Torsion and compression with loads at the same time makes torque forces.) This torque force would be the equivalent of loading the spine with over 1000 newtons, and some researchers have measured IDP as high as 4000 newtons or the equivalent of lifting about 400 lbs. over the shoulders. Forces applied to the spine such as bending, twisting, pulling and/or lifting at the same time are probably the highest forces that can be applied to the spine. These forces can contribute to back injuries. In other words, the torque and shearing forces are the culprit of most low back injuries. Examples of extreme shear loading and torque forces can occur from a high-velocity motor vehicle collision (possibly higher than thirty-five to forty-five miles per hour), particularly if the patient wears a seat belt. Segmental instability eventually causes the supporting anatomical structures to give way because these structures have been subject to stressful anatomical conditions for some time. These and other spinal abnormalities may predispose a person to develop spinal problems at different times in their lives.

The mechanics of the spine, posture, and other physical activities should be carefully assessed when one refers to "work limitations." That is why physical therapy should also be tailored to the patient's low back condition, as well as the structure, gender, shape, and constitution of the person. Recommendations for physical activities and therapy should have scientific, practical, efficient, and beneficial applications.

Some people are more prone to spinal deterioration and can therefore incur injuries to the spine far earlier than others who are performing the same activities. Similarly structured individuals may not tolerate the same physical strain as well as other persons who have different genetic backgrounds. The tissues may be more elastic and resilient in some people. Males and females also have different physical characteristics. Children typically have more elasticity, so the tissues heal easily. In contrast, adult tissues are more rigid and less resilient and the tissues tend to break more easily. As we age, the tissues tend to have less water content. Because of this, the tissues tend to break easily. Certain studies have indicated that significant axial loads over the lumbar spine will not necessarily rupture an intervertebral disc.

Many sports activities contribute to a high incidence of joint, bone, and spinal problems. As young people participate in these sports activities, many have dreams of becoming an idol or a star athlete. Of course, there is nothing wrong with having dreams as long as the young dreamer is aware that glory does have a downside—the occurrence of painful musculoskeletal conditions during young adulthood that may be carried throughout a lifetime.

Certain medical conditions occur at a relatively young age, such as bone fractures, dislocations, and soft tissue injuries (ligaments, tendons, muscle tears, and so forth). It is quite common for the young athlete to develop chronic neck pain or LBP. Surgery and postsurgical chronic pain are the norm—at a young age—for the sports person and the professional athlete.

Athletes have an especially different array of sports-related injuries. In the older population, some tissues lose certain proteins and water content. This situation causes the tissues to become hard. Thus, they do not easily regenerate.

Older people are more prone to sustain sports-related injuries. In fact, it is typical that people in their thirties or forties will try to do the same physical activities as when they were younger. Their tissues cannot withstand the same degree of physical stress (as in karate, football, and boxing) because they lack elasticity (resilience); therefore, they sustain low back injuries.

There are certain times of the day and days of the week when athletes sustain more injuries. For instance, during the first hours of the day, the discs are more hydrated, and, as the intradiscal pressures increase when bending, twisting, and lifting, it is more probable the disc will herniate or rupture in young patients.

It is in the latter part of the week when some people "have the time" to exercise and make up for past sedentary days or weeks. They engage in strenuous physical activities and injure themselves. I call this phenomenon "the make up weekend workout." Another situation is the "weekend's low back syndrome." This involves people that are out of physical condition and try to do home chores and yard work. They exert themselves doing heavy lifting, bending, and digging. These activities can hurt the lower back and rupture discs in the spine. People think they can still do the same activities they did twenty years ago with the "I am still young" attitude.

However, professional or more serious athletes may slow down on the weekend and, on the first part of the week, are back to their routines. These people have to "warm up" to avoid soft tissue injuries due to the nature and intensity of their training. Some studies of disc mechanics indicate axial loads on the spine are well-tolerated. However, rotation and flexion increase intradiscal pressure (shear forces) significantly and may account for disc ruptures.

One of the sports associated with the most cervical fractures and other injuries is football. Other full-contact activities such as karate, kickboxing, boxing, hockey, motocross, skydiving, surfing, ice-skating, waterskiing, wrestling, golfing, basketball, baseball, gymnastics, rodeo activities, and so forth are associated with multiple injuries that affect the neck, lower back, head, and so forth. As part of rigorous training in order to excel against other competitors, the athlete can often be injured. Although I do not intend to criticize any particular sport, I do want to make the young population aware of the dangers of engaging in certain sports, such as those described previously. Mechanical and biophysical principles are also in direct relationship to the patient's age, gender, weight, size, anatomical structure, and genetics when considering low back injuries.

Heavy labor and jobs requiring manly force also contribute to the grinding and eventual wearing and tearing of the body. The areas of the body most affected are the spine and the large joints such as hips, knees, and ankles. Other body parts affected by repetitive use or by resisting heavy loads are wrists, hips, and shoulders. It is typical that large people, especially men, do heavier physical tasks that are usually even more strenuous in proportion to their size. These people get hurt frequently. I call it the "Hulk's syndrome."

In order to avoid any further philosophical, social, or political analysis, I will summarize by making one final observation: Wearing and tearing will eventually claim its victim.

Brief Description of Medical Specialties

There is a tendency to confuse the functions of the different specialties in medicine. Confusion tends to create frustration on the part of patients and physicians, and it can lead to the waste of time and resources. I believe it is important patients understand basic concepts about LBP so that they can participate in decision-making processes. During their evaluation and treatment, patients should distinguish the differences among the different medical specialties.

In certain instances, the layperson does not know the fine line separating certain medical specialties. Although there are flow charts or guidelines to follow for the diagnosis and treatment of the patient with LBP, there is still some confusion pertaining to the diagnosis and treatment of patients with LBP. In some cases, general practitioners follow these flowcharts to the letter. This practice may result in wasted resources. These flowcharts are only guidelines to assist the physician, who ultimately has the last word in making a diagnosis and providing treatment. On the other hand, if a reputable journal makes a rule out of some studies, insurance companies and then physicians tend to follow the same rule. Sometimes, these publications lack prospective studies, or they generalize their concepts so they lack validity.

Certain specialties also overlap and create some confusion, for instance, neurology and neurosurgery, orthopedic surgery and rheumatology, physiatry (physical medicine and rehabilitation) and occupational medicine and industrial medicine, psychology (no MD degree) and psychiatry (MD degree), and so forth.

This topic requires a more in-depth discussion in order to explain the functions and differences among specialties. Quite often, the individual does not know the extent of the different specialties and their functions.

The following are common specialties that treat patients who have spinal problems: neurosurgery, orthopedic surgery, physiatry, neurology, occupational medicine or industrial medicine, anesthesiology (pain management), primary care physicians (family practice), and chiropractors. Each specialty plays a role in the patient's LBP management.

I will mention some of the medical specialties that could be involved in the treatment of a patient with LBP. I will also give an overview of the training required, the duration of the training, and some of their functions.

Surgical specialties:

- Neurosurgery
- Orthopedic Surgery (with a subspecialty in spine)

Nonsurgical specialties:

- Neurology
- Physiatry or Physical Medicine and Rehabilitation (PM&R)
- Anesthesia
- Occupational Medicine or Industrial Medicine
- Pain Management Specialists
- Family Practice
- Internal Medicine
- Psychiatry
- Doctors of Osteopathic Medicine

Nonphysician clinicians and licensed health care professionals:

- Doctors of Chiropractic
- Psychology
- Physician Assistant
- Nurse Practitioner
- Physical Therapist
- Occupational Therapist
- Medical Assistant

Neurosurgery. The neurosurgical residency averages five to six years after medical school. There are fellowships for specific training such as brain surgery, vascular surgery, skull base surgery, spinal surgery, and so forth. Fellowships typically are tailored to last six to twelve months after completing a full residency in the specialty.

This specialty is related to the diagnosis and surgical treatment of conditions pertaining to the central nervous system (CNS) and peripheral nervous system, including spine and nerves. Contrary to neurology, neurosurgery is related to the surgery of neurological conditions, such as brain tumors, vascular abnormalities, hydrocephalus (excessive fluid in the brain), peripheral nerves, epilepsy (including functional neurosurgery), and spinal conditions (such as tumors, vascular abnormalities, infections, degenerative diseases, and trauma).

This specialty also includes alternative surgical procedures for other painful conditions. Some neurosurgeons may implement pain management using spinal stimulators, morphine pump implants, vertebroplasty and kyphoplasty, spinal injections, and so forth. There are other applications in neurosurgery as well, such as brain stereotactic surgery for Parkinson's disease, movement disorders, trigeminal neuralgia, radiosurgery, gamma knife, and so on.

Orthopedic Surgery. The residency in this specialty averages five to six years after medical school. Some residency programs train the surgeon in spine surgery; otherwise, a spinal fellowship of six to twelve months may be taken at the end of the residency.

In this specialty, the physician treats medical problems related to the bones and joints ("bone doctor") as well as soft tissues (muscles, tendons, etc.). These physicians usually perform surgery of the bones, tendons, ligaments, and joints.

Some orthopedic surgeons have received additional training in order to treat spinal conditions such as scoliosis and spine deformities. Sometimes, these surgeons will overlap their work with neurosurgery because they have also been trained to treat degenerative spine problems (for example, spinal stenosis, herniated disc, and so forth). However, many orthopedic surgeons do not perform surgery of the spinal cord, while most neurosurgeons do perform this type of surgery. Frequently, neurosurgeons and orthopedic surgeons work hand in hand because the neurosurgeon is typically more familiar with disorders of the CNS and the use of the operating microscope for fine nerve or spinal cord conditions (for instance, spinal tumor).

Orthopedic Surgeon (subspecialty in sports-related injuries). This is a specialty in which an orthopedic surgeon completes another year of training, or fellowship, specifically in sports-related injuries. This orthopedic surgeon, compared to a sports medicine specialist, can perform surgical procedures for injuries related to sports.

Sports Medicine Specialist. In this specialty, a residency of three to five years after medical school is required. Some general practitioners receive special training in treating patients with sports-related injuries. These sports medicine specialists administer a conservative approach to treatment, and they do not perform surgery. If surgery is required for bone, joint, or soft tissues injuries, they will send the patient to a general orthopedic surgeon or an orthopedic surgeon with a subspecialty in sports medicine. Another important area of sports medicine is related to the study of body anatomy, anthropometrics, metabolic body function, and calculations for endurance and performance when engaging in sports.

Neurology. After medical school and one year of internal medicine, the residency in this specialty averages four years. A neurologist does not perform surgery of the CNS; however, they may perform some invasive procedures such as spinal taps, muscle or nerve biopsies, and EMG/NCV studies. Sometimes, a neurologist will develop pain management techniques and will learn to perform more invasive procedures.

A neurologist typically treats patients with non-surgical disorders of the CNS, such as epilepsy, stroke, movement disorders, peripheral nerve degenerative disorders (for example, MS), headaches, etc. In some instances, when surgery may be required to treat certain types of epilepsy, the neurologist will refer the patient to a neurosurgeon. Some neurologists will also administer conservative treatment in the management of LBP, and they sometimes perform independent medical evaluations (IME) and impairment ratings (IR). They also order tests for patients with LBP and neurological disorders; however, they usually refer the patient with a surgical condition to the neurosurgeon or spine surgeon.

Physiatry (Physical Medicine and Rehabilitation or PM&R). Residency in this specialty averages three to four years after medical school. It is a specialty in which the physician receives special training in the area of physical medicine and rehabilitation. The physician is usually required to complete one year of internal medicine before beginning the actual residency in PM&R.

The physician is trained in the treatment of muscles, bones and joints, soft tissue injuries, and wound care. The physician is also trained to rehabilitate patients with disabling medical conditions (for example, stroke, diabetes and paralysis). Physiatry primarily focuses on the rehabilitation of the patient. Physiatrists can perform evaluations for disability and can dictate a program of rehabilitation and treatment for the patient with "disorders of the soft tissues" as well as the CNS, which have caused deformity, contractures, and brain dysfunction. They usually work closely with physical, occupational, and speech therapists.

A physiatrist can also be involved in sports medicine, pain management, workers' compensation evaluations, and conservative treatment techniques. During the last ten years, physiatrists have become more aggressive in the treatment of patients with LBP. They sometimes perform invasive procedures such as spinal taps (epidural injections), radiofrequency treatments, nerve blocks, discograms, intradiscal electrothermal therapy (IDET), spinal stimulators, morphine pump implants, vertebroplasty, and some other spinal implants when they practice pain management (pain clinic). It is usually recommended they have the support of a spine surgeon in order to deal with possible complications.

They are often trained to perform electromyography (EMG), nerve conduction velocity (NCV) studies, and some other minimally invasive procedures. A physiatrist can perform the functions of an occupational medicine physician, and he or she can perform IME, IRE, and so forth. They can submit depositions in certain legal cases. In many instances, they will testify in court in order to establish the level of impairment that a patient has because of his or her soft tissue and bone (musculoskeletal) injuries.

Occupational Medicine or Industrial Medicine. After medical school, the average residency or training period in this specialty is three years. This is a specialty in which the physician conservatively treats patients who have work-related injuries, and the physician can perform IMEs and IRs. They not only treat patients with soft tissue injuries and nonsurgical fractures, but they can also evaluate and treat any disorder that is work-related, such as exposure to chemicals.

These physicians also evaluate working conditions, ergo dynamics at work, and OSHA regulations. They also make statistical calculations. In addition, their specialty includes preventive medicine, vaccinations, physical examinations, audiometric assessments, and pulmonary evaluations for people who work in areas where there is exposure to fumes, gases, and other chemicals. There is a special educational program for this specialty; however, some other specialties do overlap. Physicians specializing in physiatry, neurology, general surgery, orthopedic surgery, and family practice with special training can also practice occupational medicine.

Occupational medicine physicians are trained to identify forms of chemical and physical exposure. The occupational medicine physician regularly performs annual and preadmission physical exams as well as basic blood work for toxins, urine tests, drug screening, vaccinations, working condition evaluations and other studies. They also can perform audiological and visual evaluations.

Anesthesiology. The residency in this specialty averages three to four years after medical school. During the residency, physicians learn the techniques and proper use of different medications in order to anesthetize a patient who typically requires surgery or other painful procedures. Some anesthesiologists especially prefer to treat patients with chronic painful medical conditions, and they typically run pain clinics. These physicians are more oriented to the use of analgesics for pain control.

Pain Management Specialist. There is an American Board of Pain Management. Certain physicians who treat painful conditions—such as anesthesiologists, physiatrists, neurologists, neurosurgeons, orthopedic surgeons, and general practitioners—can apply for the certification relating to this specialty. There is no residency program for this rapidly evolving branch of medicine. In fact, any physician with some basic knowledge of certain injections and pain management techniques can practice this branch of medicine without necessarily being board certified by the American Academy of Pain Management (AAPM).

To be certified by the AAPM, one must register as a member, take certain courses, and comply with their exam requirements. During these courses, a physician must master the use of narcotic pain medications and must become familiar with the laws and regulations related to the use of narcotics and other pain medications. The practitioner is trained to use invasive procedures such as spinal stimulators and pump implants. A physician is encouraged to learn other pain management techniques as well.

Typically, these specialists treat patients who have painfully chronic, disabling medical conditions. Through seminars, hands-on courses (usually on cadavers), and examinations, a physician can become board certified in pain management. These programs train a physician to develop different pain management techniques using pain medications, combinations of medications, doses of medications, etc. Physicians can be trained to perform minimally invasive procedures such as the insertion of morphine pumps and spinal stimulators. Some of these "minimally invasive procedures" can lead to devastating complications that could cause permanent disability. It is highly recommended that physicians who are practicing pain management have the support and backup of a spine surgeon who is trained and willing to address potentially serious complications.

Family Practice. The residency in family practice lasts three years after medical school. Physicians are trained to extend their knowledge in general medicine, including internal medicine, surgery, pediatrics, and obstetrics/gynecology.

Internal Medicine. Following medical school, the residency takes about three years to complete. Physicians are trained to treat patients with disorders of the internal organs. Sometimes, there are subspecialties such as pulmonology, neurology, gastroenterology, and others.

Psychiatry. Following medical school, the residency takes approximately three to four years to complete. In addition, one year of internal medicine is required to join the residency program. These physicians perform psychiatric evaluations and treatment of patients with mental illnesses. A psychiatrist is a medical doctor who completes an average of five years of residency in the specialty after medical school. A psychologist does not hold a medical degree.

Doctor of Osteopathy (DO). The average time to complete the doctorate in osteopathic medicine degree is four to five years. A DO attends a medical school that is similar to other medical schools. They receive training and medical education as well as some chiropractic management, which includes bone and joint manipulations. A DO can complete a residency program in a specialty.

Other Nonphysician Health Care Providers or Health Care Allied Practitioners

Nonphysician clinicians and licensed health care professionals include (but are not limited to): chiropractors, nurse practitioners, physician's assistants, physical therapists, occupational therapists, and psychologists.

Chiropractor or DC (Doctor of Chiropractic). The average length of time to complete this program is three to four years, and there is no need to attend medical school. Chiropractors diagnose and treat certain medical conditions based mainly on the patient's history and exam, but they usually do not conduct any lab studies other than X-rays. However, in some settings, a chiropractor can order CT and MRI scans, but they cannot prescribe medications. They primarily focus their treatment on manipulations of the spine because they correlate medical problems with the spinal column and the central nervous system. However, they may use other techniques to treat patients such as herbal remedies, massage, acupressure, and so forth. Chiropractors cannot enter a residency in a medical specialty.

Psychology. There is no need for a medical degree. These people or health care allied practitioners cannot prescribe medications. They can only perform psychological evaluations and sometimes provide counseling in certain settings.

Physician's Assistant (PA). After high school, the average length of time to complete this program is two to three years. A PA has completed special training in the use of diagnostic tools that can assess a patient's condition. The PA can assist the physician in the evaluation and treatment of a patient; however, they are required to be under the supervision of a medical doctor and are often not allowed to prescribe medications in some states. The PA can relieve the physician of many cumbersome duties so that the physician can focus on the evaluation and treatment of the patient. PAs are not required to obtain a medical degree.

Certified Nurse Practitioner (CNP). The average length of time to complete this program is three to four years following nursing school. CNPs are trained in several aspects of medical practice, including obtaining a medical history, examining the patient, diagnosing and treating the patient, and occasionally prescribing medications (with or without the physician's supervision, according to state laws). They may also supervise other practitioners such as medical assistants (CMA, if certified), nurse's aides (CNA, if certified), and other personnel. (BSN: bachelor of science degree in nursing) (MSN: master of science degree in nursing).

Medical Assistant (MA)/Certified Medical Assistant (CMA). This program requires approximately eight months of schooling. An MA is trained to obtain a medical history and records, record vital signs, assist in minor surgery, remove sutures, change dressing from wounds, and call in prescriptions (with the physician's authorization). They also learn to draw blood, prepare patients for exam, explain treatment and diagnosis to the patient, update medical records, make appointments for patients, and file insurance forms. An MA learns to perform several functions in a doctor's office including the front desk, for example, appointments, referrals, and so on.

Nurse Assistant (NA)/Nurse's aide. The average training program is one year. They are trained to assist nurses, and they assist in transferring, transporting, bathing, and grooming patients. In addition, they aid patients in performing range-of-motion exercises, and they record patient information.

Physical Therapist (PT)/Occupational Therapist (OT). This program requires two to three years of schooling. A physical therapist treats patients who require rehabilitation by assisting them in performing specific exercises and providing other modes of therapy.

In this segment of Chapter One, I have outlined several of the school programs and the training requirements for some of the most common medical specialties as well as the requirements for the health care allied practitioners. Some programs vary in the length of time that is necessary to complete them, and they vary in the method of teaching.

The extent of training and the capabilities of these specialties are not carved in stone. Their functions may overlap. Although there is a basic training period for these specialties during residency, certain occupations do not have specific boundaries. Not every specialist can perform certain procedures that care for patients with LBP. A neurologist or a physiatrist (or any other nonsurgical specialist), for instance, would not be expected to perform brain or spine surgery.

The specific program and training requirements for the various specialties and for the health care allied practitioners may vary from state to state and from school to school. I recommend that any person interested in knowing more about current program requirements contact the appropriate agencies and schools in order to receive more specific and accurate information.

Questions

Which specialist do I need to see? A patient with LBP, generally speaking, should see a spine surgeon if the pain was severe from the beginning and has lingered for more than two weeks. If there is LBP associated with pain and numbness in the legs and/or other neurological deficits such as weakness or bladder or rectal dysfunction, the patient should go to the local emergency room for medical evaluation. Emergency surgery may be required.

Certain specialists are capable of treating patients with LBP, including neurosurgeons, orthopedic surgeons, general practitioners (family practitioners), occupational medicine specialists, sports medicine specialists, neurologists, physiatrists, as well as the other physicians and health care allied practitioners I have already mentioned in this chapter. It is likely a spine surgeon will provide a more definitive treatment plan and will direct the patient to the appropriate specialist, if surgery is not warranted.

Whose recommendations should I follow: my primary physician or the secondary surgical opinion? If the patient requires spine surgery or treatment for LBP, then the patient should strongly consider the recommendations made by the spine surgeon. Although the primary care physician's intent is for the patient to receive the best possible medical care, he or she does not have the training necessary to recognize specific problems of the spine for which a patient may need surgery.

CHAPTER 2

Causes of LBP

When patients ask me this question, I tell them there are several causes of LBP. Patients think of only a few causes of LBP such as "pulled muscles" or a "slipped disc." People tend to assume a ruptured disc is the only and most likely cause of back pain. I have made a list of causes of LBP. Many of the causes of LBP are uncommon, but I have included a long list. LBP can be related to any of the anatomical structures in the lower back. In some cases, LBP can radiate to the legs. Disorders of internal organs can be associated with LBP. Wear and tear of the bones, cartilage (discs), tendons, and muscles (degenerative disease) are associated with LBP in several occasions.

LBP may or may not be associated with leg pain. When LBP is associated with leg pain, compression of the nerve or sciatica may be suspected ("pinched nerve"). However, leg pain is not always related to a herniated disc. There are many other causes of leg pain not associated with LBP.

The reader will find words and terms in this chapter that are difficult to understand because of their technicality. I recommend the layperson pay special attention to the most frequent causes of LBP. I have included long lists of causes of LBP that involve medical terms. This book is intended to assist not only the layperson but also the person with some medical background. In general, frequent causes of LBP are poor posture (body mechanics) and chronic stress to the ligaments, tendons, and muscles in the lower back. The cause of LBP in as much as eighty percent is impossible to accurately diagnose. However, some researchers believe the cause of eighty percent of all LBP is strained muscles. A high percentage of people with LBP have an arthritic origin.

I classified causes of LBP by:

- Frequency in general
- Age group
- Organ and systems
- LBP associated with leg pain

- Leg pain with and without LBP
- Main causes of leg pain without LBP
- Confusing diagnosis
- Special entities that can be related to LBP and/or leg pain (fibromyalgia, myofascial pain, chronic fatigue syndrome, depression, stress-related illnesses, irritable bowel syndrome, and so forth)

The most frequent causes of LBP (LBP) in general are:

- Mechanical problems such as obesity, poor body ergonomics, and posture. Prolonged bed rest and inactivity. (The prolonged use of back braces may make the lower back muscles weak and lead to LBP.)
- Arthritis and musculoskeletal conditions such as lumbar sprain/strain, degenerative bone and joint disease, spondylolysis, sacroiliac joint dysfunction, and fibromyalgia
- Disc herniation (and internal disc disruption)
- Spinal stenosis
- Osteoporosis
- Trauma such as contusion and fracture
- Congenital disease and spine deformities such as scoliosis, spondylolisthesis, kyphosis, spina bifida, diastematomyelia, transitional vertebra, and other variants
- Spinal instability

Causes of LBP by Age Group

- Infancy to age 20
- 20–30 years of age
- 30–50 years of age
- 50 and older

Infancy to Age 20. By far, the most frequent causes of LBP in this group age are events related to the musculoskeletal system. These are some of the most frequent causes of LBP in this group are:

- Sprain/strain
- Heavy exertion (athletes)
- Heavy work

- Disc herniation
- Congenital spine abnormalities (vascular malformations, congenital tumors, dysrhaphism, spinal bifida, tethered spinal cord, myelomeningocele, lipoma, and so forth)

Disc herniation tends to be underdiagnosed in children. Because of the resilience and the still-growing capacity of the tissues, children usually heal spontaneously with no surgery. Some studies revealed more children with disc herniations than previously thought.

There are four major types of deformity of the spine (see the illustrations at the end of this chapter):

1) Kyphosis is a deformity of the spine in which the patient tends to crouch or bend the spine forward.

2) Scoliosis is a deformity of the spine sideways.

3) Lordosis is an exaggeration of the normal curvature of the spine.

4) Spondylolisthesis is slippage of the vertebral bones one over another, and spondylolysis is the breaking down of a vertebra.

Other less frequent causes of LBP in childhood and adolescence can be:

- Congenital defects
- Vascular malformation (vascular anomalies including epidural varicose perineural veins, postoperative neovascular malformations, AVMs, and variants of vascular malformations) Some of these entities are not yet clearly described in medical textbooks.
- Tumor
- Infections such as urinary tract infections, bone infections, and viral infections
- Trauma
- Leukemia
- Sickle cell disease
- Hereditary rheumatoid arthritis
- Rheumatic fever
- Referred pain
- Psychological
- Other (vascular anomalies and malformations with or without previous surgery). **Syndrome of the Taut Ligament.** It is a lateral recess syndrome

related to a vertical, taut ligamentum flavum pressing the nerve root as it runs through the lateral recess. It is frequently associated with congenital shortened pedicles. This is a new entity not yet published in textbooks or journals, as far as I know. It is a syndrome and an anatomical variant. It is an operative finding the author has noticed in some patients.

Young adults (20–30 years)

- Sprain/Strain (sports-related and work-related)
- Poor posture
- Heavy exertion
- Trauma
- Disc herniation
- Viral infections
- Psychological
- Congenital abnormalities
- Other

Adults (30–50 years)

- Postural
- Sprain/Strain (work-related)
- Referred pain (organ-related)
- Trauma
- Psychological (secondary gain)
- Infections (flu-like syndrome)
- Disc herniation
- Failed back surgery (patient with chronic LBP after one or more surgical procedures)
- Osteoarthritis and other types of joint disease
- Facet joint syndrome
- Fibromyalgia
- RSD and leg pain
- Spinal stenosis
- Cancer (tumor)
- Mechanical (postural pain and obesity)

Adults 50 and older

- Osteoarthritis and other joint disease
- Spinal stenosis
- Degenerative disc and bone disease
- Herniated disc
- Sprain/Strain
- Failed back surgery (patient with chronic LBP after one or more surgical procedures)
- Infections (flu-like syndrome)
- Cancer
- Referred organ or system pain
- Facet joint syndrome
- RSD and leg pain

Causes of LBP by Organ and Body System

- Joint and musculoskeletal disorders
- Psychological
- Mass lesions (benign and malignant)
- Infectious
- Neurological
- Hematological
- Vascular
- Endocrinological
- Mechanical pain (postural)
- Systemic and related to internal organs (referred pain)

Joint and musculoskeletal conditions that cause LBP can be classified as follows:

- Sprain/strain (such as the ones related to post-seizure state, athletic, piriformis muscle syndrome, heavy exertion and work)
- Osteoarthritis (commonly known by the layperson as "arthritis") and osteoarthrosis
- Fibromyalgia

- **Facet joint syndrome.** This is a term not clearly understood, but it is thought to be inflammation or degenerative changes of the joint for any cause, such as whiplash injuries, osteoarthritis, and so forth.
- Sacroiliac joint dysfunction
- Connective tissue diseases such as lupus, rheumatoid arthritis (RA), ankylosing spondylitis (AS), scleroderma, dermatomyositis, polymyositis/dermatomyositis (combination of both), polymyalgia rheumatica, spondylosis and degenerative bone and disc disease (osteophytes known as "bone spurs"), Reiter's syndrome, psoriasis, Behçet's syndrome, enteropathic arthritis, Whipple's disease, hydradenitis suppurative, polyarteritis nodosa, or arthritic process of the sacroiliac joints and/or hips
- Fibrositis
- Chronic fatigue syndrome
- Spondylolisthesis (stable and unstable)
- Spondylolysis, kyphosis, lordosis, and deformity of the spine (acquired or congenital)
- Rheumatic fever
- Familial Mediterranean fever
- Diffuse idiopathic skeletal hyperostosis (DISH)
- Osteitis condensans Ilii
- Porphyria
- Lipids disorder
- Paget's disease
- OPLL or ossification of the posterior longitudinal ligament
- OLF or ossification of the ligamentum flavum
- Bone cyst or hemangioma
- Pathological fracture (as in cancer)
- Osteogenesis imperfecta
- Hereditary bone deformities or malformations
- Medication-related LBP
- Transitional vertebra, long transverse process and other anatomical variations
- Ileotransverse ligament syndrome

- Marfan's syndrome
- Spina Bifida Occulta, dysrhaphism, myelomeningocele, lipoma, tethered spinal cord, and so forth

Psychological disorders include:

- Depression
- Anxiety
- Secondary gain (disability), need of attention, monetary compensation, malingering, and so forth
- Hysteria, psychosis, neurosis, hallucinations, and other psychiatric entities
- Personality disorders (obsessive/compulsive disorder, hypochondrias, and so forth)
- Munchausen's syndrome.
- Narcotic or drug addiction (drug-seeking behavior personality)

Mass lesions can be benign and malignant. There can be tumors and invasive lesions of the lumbosacral spine including benign cystic lesions.

- Multiple myeloma
- Bone metastases
- Lymphoma
- Intraspinal tumors (Lipoma with or without tethered spinal cord, Meningioma, schwannoma, neurofibroma, ependymoma, medulloblastoma, astrocytoma, hemangioma, pseudogout, synovial cyst)
- Osteoid osteoma
- Chondroma and chondrosarcoma
- Osteoblastoma
- Giant cell tumor
- Hemangioma or bone angioma
- Eosinophilic granuloma
- Sacroiliac lipomata
- Aneurysmal bone cyst
- Arachnoid cyst
- Gaucher's disease
- Chordoma

- Leukemia
- Epidural lipomatosis
- Amyloidosis and Sarcoidosis
- Nerve tumor

Infectious processes

- Vertebral osteomyelitis
- Intervertebral disc infection
- Pyogenic sacroiliitis
- Herpes Zoster (Shingles). May mimic LBP or other soft tissue (muscle) or bone/joint pain.
- Paget's disease of the bone
- Tuberculosis (Pot's disease with bone destruction)
- Fungus infections
- Meningitis
- Spine abscess
- Abscess and compression of peripheral nerves
- Parasitic infestation (trichinosis, cysticercosis) with direct infiltration of the muscles
- AIDS
- Tetanus
- Typhoid fever
- Dengue (breakbone fever)
- Influenza and other wintry, flu-like syndromes
- Tick fever
- Rabies
- Rift Valley Fever
- Rickettsioses
- Q Fever
- Lyme disease
- Other less frequent infections

Neurogenic entities

- Syringomyelia

- Parkinson's disease
- Motor tics and other movement disorders that can cause chronic strains and sprains
- Dystonia
- Thalamic syndrome and other painful neurological conditions
- Multiple sclerosis (MS)
- Amyotrophic lateral sclerosis (ALS)
- Dystonic and extrapyramidal reactions to sickness and adverse reactions to medications
- Muscle contractures related to neurological disorders and medication-related syndromes
- Diabetic neuropathy
- Hypokalemia and other electrolytic and hormonal unbalances

There are medical entities that are distinguished more for muscle weakness rather than for pain. However, some of these entities may start with muscle weakness and later, during the course of the diseased, they may cause some degree of muscle aching and pain.

Hematological (related to blood disorders) can be associated with LBP:

- Myelofibrosis
- Hemoglobinopathies, paroxysmal nocturnal hemoglobinuria (associated sometimes with mesenteric and hepatic vein thrombosis)
- Hemophilia related to bruising and hemorrhage
- Sickle cell disease
- Spherocytosis (associated with cholecystitis)
- Splenomegaly
- Hemolytic anemia
- Thrombotic thrombocytopenic purpura (associated with pancreatitis)

Vascular conditions

- Arterial venous malformation (AVM) and other vascular anomalies, including epidural varicose perineural veins (a new entity not yet described in some medical textbooks). There can be postoperative neovascular formations, malformations, and AVMs that can be related to LBP and/or leg pain.
- Abdominal aortic aneurysm and peripheral vascular ischemic disease

- Hemorrhage (spinal subdural or extradural hematoma and subarachnoid hemorrhage)
- Hematoma (blood clots related to trauma or spontaneous hemorrhage) of the soft tissues with or without compression of peripheral nerves can cause LBP and/or leg pain.

There can be endocrinologic, metabolic, poisons, and other systemic disorders related to LBP, including:

- Osteoporosis
- Pituitary disease (and electrolytic imbalance)
- Cushing's syndrome and Cushing's disease (electrolytic imbalance)
- Ochronosis
- Gout (uric acid disorder)
- Osteomalacia and hormone-related diseases (parathyroid disorders occurring with calcium and phosphorus imbalances)
- Microcrystalline disease
- Diabetes with peripheral neuropathy
- Obesity
- Smoking (it has been associated with osteoporosis)
- Alcoholism with chronic calcium, phosphorus, electrolytic or hormonal imbalance and with vitamin deficiency
- Thyroid and parathyroid disorders
- Drugs related to adverse reactions to certain medications
- Poison (strychnine), PCP, tetanus, black widow spider bite, heat stroke, and so forth
- Porphyria (cholelithiasis)
- Alkaptonuria
- Hyperlipoproteinemia (hepatosplenomegaly)
- Chromosomal or Genetic: Dwarfism, Turner's syndrome, and so forth
- Acromegaly
- Osteopetrosis
- Renal osteodystrophy
- Electrolytic and metabolic imbalance, specifically the ones related with calcium, phosphorus, magnesium, and potassium

- Vitamin D-resistant rickets (VDRR)
- Cirrhosis and other liver disorders

These are other causes of LBP, including the following mechanical deformities:

- Scoliosis
- Degenerative disc disease (with or without bulging or herniated disc)
- Spinal stenosis
- Spondylolysis
- Spondylolisthesis (with or without instability)
- Overweight/Obesity
- Pregnancy and increased lordosis of the lumbar spine
- Poor posture in general
- Failed back surgery syndrome (with and without hardware implant). There is pain related to scar tissue from back surgery (arachnoiditis, epidural scar, and discitis). There is pain associated with placement of hardware (plates and screws or other hardware) for spinal fusion.
- Flat back syndrome (commonly associated with surgery and placement of Harrington rods)
- Lumbar (lumbosacral) instability from trauma, congenital, iatrogenic (as a complication after surgery), and degenerative
- Prolonged bed rest and poor sleeping habits
- Deformity of the lower back by awkward or bizarre postures (psychological, use of crutches, prosthesis, bad habits, and so forth)
- Prolonged sitting, driving, or standing

Large breasts in women can be the cause of upper back pain that can transmit to the lower back by changing and altering the mechanics of the lower back spine.

- Referred pain arises from a certain internal organ, but the pain is reflected in a distant part of the body. These are some organ and system-related causes of LBP:
- Retroperitoneal fibrosis
- Sarcoidosis
- Gastrointestinal problems related to conditions of the esophagus (hiatal hernia, cancer, esophagitis), duodenum (ulcer), stomach (ulcer, gastritis, cancer), pancreas (inflammation, cancer), colon (diverticulitis, ulcera-

tive colitis, cancer), gallbladder (inflammation, tumor), and liver (cirrhosis and inflammation as in hepatitis and tumor)

- Genitourinary disorders related to the kidney (infections such as pyelonephritis and stones in the urinary tract), ureter (hydronephrosis and hydronephritis), bladder (infection, chronic inflammation, tumor), prostate (infection, tumor), female genital organs (pelvic inflammatory disease), uterus (endometriosis, endometritis, postpartum infection, abortion), fallopian tubes (ectopic pregnancy, inflammation) and ovary (cysts, tumors)
- Aortic aneurysm
- Cancer in any of the organs of the abdomen or pelvis
- Disorders of the organs in the chest (rarely)
- Pain that originated from the genitourinary tract and from other pelvic organs is a common cause of LBP.

LBP associated with leg pain (LBP/leg pain):

- Poor posture
- Sprain/Strain
- Fibromyalgia
- Trauma
- Psychological
- Arthritic conditions
- Herniated disc
- Spinal stenosis
- Bone deformities (acquired or congenital) and spinal instability
- Facet joint syndrome
- Osteoporosis
- Chronic fatigue syndrome
- Mechanical (obesity, overweight, pregnancy)
- Tumor
- Referred pain from other organs (pancreas, stomach, duodenum, genitourinary)
- Scoliosis

- Failed back surgery
- RSD (CRPS I)
- Diabetes

There is a great difference to the physician between a patient that presents with LBP only and LBP with leg pain. There are entities that are associated with only leg pain and no LBP. How does the physician know the source of the pain? Basic knowledge of medicine will direct the physician to a most likely diagnosis. The principles of anatomy and physiology usually direct the physician to a diagnosis. We use what is called symptomatology or clinical picture, terms physicians use to gather all the symptoms patients experience to make a clinical diagnosis. (A clinical diagnosis is the one made by only using a medical history and physical exam without radiological studies, labs, or other studies.)

Then why is it so important the physician perform a thorough history and exam of the patient? A great deal of information is obtained through the history of the symptoms. When did the pain start? How long does the pain last? Is it continuous or constant? Is it intermittent? Where does the pain radiate? What are the characteristics of the pain (dull, throbbing, burning, sharp, or aching)? Does it follow a pattern? Is the pain worse in the morning or at night? Is it associated with stiffness, fever, or some other symptom? Is the pain severe, moderate, or minimal? Is it getting worse? Better? Is there any variation with the use of medications? Improvement or no change? Are there certain physical activities or positions that cause more pain or alleviate the pain? It is my experience that patients do not expect me to ask many questions about the characteristics of pain. Patients wonder why other doctors did not ask all these questions. Patients do not realize that, during the diagnosis-making process, the medical history is of paramount importance. In fact, by the time I obtained my history, I have a very good idea of what could be causing the pain even before I perform the physical exam. Some doctor's offices have questionnaires to fill out pertaining to medical history. (I do.) Other physicians have a nurse, a physician assistant, or someone else take a medical history. Description, radiation, and characteristics of the pain are key elements to making a more accurate diagnosis.

Patients refer to "sciatica" (si-at-'i-kah) when there is leg pain or LBP and leg pain. Indeed, even physicians use this term, but only when there is a well-defined pain pattern. Sciatica or sciatic pain is defined as LBP that radiates into the posterior aspect of the hip, down the leg, and below the knee. This pattern is typical true sciatic pain. However, the pain sometimes extends only to the posterior aspect of the thigh. There is no sciatic pain by definition if the pain starts in the lower back but without radiation down the leg. If the pain stays in the lower back with some discomfort in the hip, the pain is not necessarily considered "sciatica." There has been some controversy if radiation of LBP into the hip area is already considered as sciatica. The key point when defining sciatica is radiation of the pain down the leg that follows an anatomical pattern.

The exam is also extremely important, but being able to interpret the findings of the exam is more important. There are sometimes cultural and even racial features when patients describe characteristics and patterns of pain. One, as a physician, must be aware of these different cultural expressions of pain. I have consulted patients with certain cultural backgrounds that complain of leg pain when they mean knee pain or some other kind of pain. Radiation of the pain can also be difficult to interpret for the physician. Certain cultures show more emotional expression of pain than others. One of the most frequently confusing diagnoses can be hip pain with radiation down the leg. Sometimes, there is pain radiating from the hip up the lower back.

When a physician performs a physical examination on a patient with LBP, one must look for certain signs. The most frequent parts of the exam involve:

- Inspection (deformities, trauma, congenital deformities, swelling, lumps, skin changes, and so forth)
- Palpation and areas of pain or tenderness (bones, joints, lumps, and so forth)
- Range of motion of the joints (pain, stiffness, and deformity)
- Auscultation for bruits in the arteries (aneurysm, fistula, and so forth)
- Muscle strength
- Sensory exam or sensitivity
- Deep tendon reflexes (DTRs)
- Specific search for signs and certain examinations such as the straight-leg-raising (SLR) maneuver, Babinski sign, Tinel sign at the hip, and other signs (Waddell). It is recommended avoiding manipulations of the lumbar spine during the exam.
- Measurement of the length and width of the limbs. (Be aware of muscle atrophy.)
- Voluntary or involuntary movements of the extremities
- Vascular system (varicose veins, swelling, aneurysm, pulses, skin changes, skin atrophy, and so forth)
- Walking pattern
- Psychological reactions to pain, inadvertent reaction, and other emotional responses

LBP can be associated with upper back pain and with neck pain. Sometimes, it can be associated with headaches. I have treated patient who were very sensitive to pain (low pain tolerance) and experienced fainting spells or dizziness. Some others had a vagal reaction (vagal reaction refers to a manifestation of symptoms, including fainting spells, sweating, dizziness, and dropped blood pressure and pulse) associated with a painful physical experience. Visual stimuli can also trigger a vagal reaction as in the well-known reaction of fainting with the sight of blood, odors, and other stimuli. A vagal reaction is a body reaction or response of the autonomic system of the central nervous system. It is more frequent that LBP radiates up to the upper back and neck, but it is not likely that neck pain radiates down to the lower back. However, it may radiate into the upper back. Health care providers label these patients as "emotional," "hysterical," or "fakers." One must be cautious with these patients because they can have a real disorder overlapping with an "emotional" reaction. Patients sometimes take pain medication before visiting the doctor. Pain medication may mask the pain and alter the results of a medical evaluation. Patients may experience hypertension due to pain. These patients must be treated for pain and for hypertension.

Causes of leg pain:

- Hip disorders (osteoarthritis, necrosis of the femoral head, bursitis, and so forth)
- Vascular events (varicose veins, deep venous thrombosis, arterial occlusion)
- Bone and joint infections or other disorders
- Lymphatic system-related conditions
- RSD (Reflex Sympathetic Dystrophy) or CRPS I Complex Regional Pain Syndrome)
- Trauma (nerve or extremity trauma such as lesions of the nerve by sharp instruments or by gunshot and contusion of a nerve)
- Peripheral neuropathy, nerve disorders, and compressive neuropathies. Piriformis muscle syndrome is compression of the sciatic nerve on the posterior aspect of the hip (buttock). This can be related to several causes, including compression of the nerve by a wallet or other object carried in the back pocket. Meralgia paresthetica (peripheral neuropathy). Hereditary neuropathies.
- Skin-related conditions (herpes zoster/shingles and other skin disorders)

- Metabolic (imbalances of potassium, calcium, magnesium, and so forth), endocrinologic (also associated with electrolytic imbalance), and edema (swelling).
- Sciatica related to diabetes.
- Unknown neuropathies (diabetic, uremic, thyroid-related, and so forth).
- Mechanical causes (for compression of the nerves). There can be compression in the spinal canal or at the nerve itself, such as a herniated disc, spinal tumor, spinal cyst, spinal stenosis, osteoarthritis, and facet joint syndrome.
- Strain/sprain and other musculoskeletal disorders (sports-related or repetitive injury to the soft tissues)
- Restless Leg Syndrome (RLS), myoclonic disorders, twitches, dyskinesia, dystonia, muscular dystrophies, muscular contractures, Parkinson's disease, and other movement disorders usually do not cause leg pain, but they can cause some discomfort.
- Inflammation or infection of the soft tissues (cellulitis, abscess, and so forth)
- Animal bites
- Raynaud's disease and phenomenon
- Hernias (in the groin area)
- Hemorrhage or stroke (hematoma in the extremities with nerve or vascular compression)
- Compression of the nerves at the abdomen and pelvis (tumor or masses of abdominal or pelvic organs)Spinal infection (abscess)
- Cancer
- Miscellaneous (refer to some previously listed causes of LBP)
- Synovial cyst

There are entities that are difficult to diagnose. Sometimes, more than one disease or entity overlaps. Frequent causes of LBP that may become confusing for the patient and that are difficult to diagnose are outlined subsequently. In my experience, these causes of LBP and leg pain can have similar characteristics in their pattern, and they are mistakenly diagnosed frequently.

The causes of leg pain are related to the anatomical part that is affected. However, leg pain may not necessarily be related to a mechanical problem in which there is nerve compression. There can also be other nonmechanical causes of leg pain, for example, calcium, magnesium, and potassium imbalances. Some of these conditions can be associated with swelling of the leg(s). The swelling itself can cause leg pain or discomfort sometimes as in endocrinologic or metabolic disorders in which there can be fluid retention (edema). There can be leg pain related to vascular compromise (arterial or venous). Vascular compromise may involve arterial blockage (ischemic) or blood clots in the veins (thrombosis) with subsequent blockage in the blood flow return [deep venous thrombosis (DVT) and thrombophlebitis]. There can be arterial blockage with claudication (poor arterial circulation in the iliac arteries in the pelvis) with resulting leg pain. Claudication is a medical term to describe pain in the leg(s) that appears mainly when walking. Claudication can be neurogenic or vascular. It is neurogenic when there is nerve compression such as in spinal stenosis. It can be vascular when there is poor circulation (ischemia).

There are special medical conditions (for example, lymphatic system disorders) that can cause swelling of the leg(s) and sometimes pain. The symptoms and signs are relatively specific, and they have some differences when compared with each other.

Frequently Confusing Diagnoses in Patients with LBP and Leg Pain

- Hip pain, degenerative arthritis, femoral head necrosis, and bursitis
- Sacroiliac joint dysfunction (a vague term to mention pain that could be related to osteoarthritis, ankylosing spondylitis, rheumatoid arthritis, and others)
- Facet joint pain
- Peripheral vascular disease (arterial or venous)
- Peripheral neuropathy (any kind including shingles, diabetic neuropathy, alcoholic neuropathy, thyroid disease, and other conditions)
- Leg edema related to multiple causes (varicose veins, arterial or venous obstruction, angioedema, lymphedema, joint disease, hypothyroidism, renal and cardiac disease, and so forth)
- Kidney stones and (in general) any disorder of the genitourinary tract can mimic low back conditions.
- Groin hernias

It is my personal observation that some people have a hereditary tendency to have early joint and bone deterioration, including spine conditions. Contributing factors also accelerate the deterioration process, such as obesity, poor posture, heavy work, smoking, and high-impact sports and activities. It has been proven that LBP and leg pain can be caused not only by mechanical compression of the nerves. There is also a chemical irritation of the nerves by the disc content in the case of disc herniation. That is how "discogenic pain" may be explained when there is only a small- or moderate-sized bulging disc viewed on an MRI scan of the spine.

Some physicians refer to disc herniation or degenerative disc disease and a bulging disc as "leaking discs." This does not mean the disc is actively leaking material. It means the inside of the disc, the jellylike content, has bulged out from the center of the disc. The material is still contained by the fibers of ligament; however, the ruptured disc splits into one or more fragments in some instances. We call that a "free fragment" of a herniated disc. This situation has a particular significance for the physician.

There are different ways a patient with a herniated disc in the lumbar spine may present to the physician. Some patients have only LBP. Others have only leg pain. But the majority of patients with a herniated disc have both LBP and leg pain. The MRI scan can be confusing for some patients and even for some physicians. I have examined patients with a herniated disc on one side, but the patient has pain on the opposite side. I have seen patients with a small disc herniation causing severe pain and patients with a large disc herniation causing only moderate or minimal pain. Patients with a disc herniation may present with only leg pain and no numbness or weakness. Others have numbness and no pain. Less frequently, some patients can complain of weakness in the leg(s) but no pain or numbness. Patients with a disc herniation present with LBP, leg pain, numbness, and/or weakness in the leg(s) most frequently. I have seen patients who improve right after surgery and others who continue to experience leg pain. The lingering leg pain is usually related to the prolonged time the nerve was compressed although this is not necessarily true. Each patient can present with a different clinical picture, and not all patients with the same conditions are treated the same way. There are clear-cut cases in which surgery is mandatory, and there is a standard treatment for these medical conditions.

I would like to comment on the so-called "facet joint syndrome." There is controversy in the medical literature, and some books even describe different symptoms and signs between "facet joint syndrome," disc herniation, and other entities such as spinal stenosis. It is my opinion there are patients who do have pain originating in the joints and cause, to some extent, symptoms and signs similar to the ones with disc herniation. There are some differences, however, in the clinical presentation. Patients whose pain originates in the joints tend to have pain that is localized precisely to the area of the joints. Frequently, patients feel or hear a "pop" when they have an onset of back pain. However, the "pop" is not typical of facet pain. The pain tends to radiate across the lower back and down to one leg or another or sometimes (less frequently) to both legs, but the pain tends to radiate no further down than the knee level. Other characteristics can be investigated in the exam. I do not consider this is a book in which I can describe medical terminology for the diagnosis of certain conditions such as this. Therefore, I will not dwell upon this entity in this book.

Special Entities as a Cause of LBP with and without Leg Pain

I think I should comment on medical entities that are frequently confused with each other. It is known that people form support groups and associations to deal with poorly understood disorders. Books and extensive literature have been written on these syndromes and disorders.

We refer to a group of symptoms and signs in medicine as a "syndrome." Usually, there is no clear cause of symptoms. (There are usually theories of causes of a syndrome.) Syndromes are still under investigation for the cause, diagnosis, and treatment. Usually, a newly discovered entity in medicine is called a syndrome while research reveals the cause of the symptoms and signs. When we learn more about a syndrome (such as the cause, natural history, and the treatment), we call it a disease or disorder. Some of these disorders and syndromes are:

- Non-Osteoarthritis and Non-Rheumatoid Arthritis Syndrome (NONRAS)
- Fibromyalgia (FM)
- Myofascial pain (MPS)
- Chronic fatigue syndrome (CFS)
- Depression (several levels of depression)
- Irritable bowel syndrome (IBS)
- Reflex Sympathetic Dystrophy (RSD) or Complex Regional Pain Syndrome (CRPS)
- Multiple chemical symptoms (MCS)/Idiopathic environmental intolerance (IEI)
- Restless Leg Syndrome

Other unusual disorders that can cause symptoms similar to the ones found in patients with chronic fatigue syndrome can be

- Epstein-Barr Virus
- Blood disorders

- Mononucleosis
- Chronic infections (including chronic hepatitis)
- Multiple sclerosis (MS)
- Chronic fungus infections
- Metal and other chemical and radioactive intoxications (uranium, plutonium, and so forth) and exposures (mercury, lead, arsenic, radon, and insecticides or pesticides)
- Vitamin deficiencies or intoxication
- Endocrinologic disorders

These are specific entities that can be diagnosed only after a meticulous and thorough medical evaluation with extensive testing.

Non-Osteoarthritis and Non-Rheumatoid Arthritis Syndrome (NON-RAS). In my practice, I have observed patients that have symptoms that do not correspond to rheumatoid arthritis or to osteoarthritis, but their symptoms overlap with each other. This syndrome is only my clinical observation.

In this syndrome, the symptoms are very similar to those seen in patients with rheumatoid arthritis yet the laboratory tests are normal. I have called this syndrome "NONRAS" (not yet described in medical textbooks under this term). The symptoms in these patients are less severe than in patients with rheumatoid arthritis. The laboratory studies are negative for lupus, ankylosing spondylitis, rheumatoid arthritis, psoriasis, or other connective tissue disorders. On the other hand, these patients have more pronounced symptoms (more incapacitating pain, joint swelling, and stiffness) than those with benign osteoarthritis. These patients are difficult to treat because they usually do not respond to medications aimed to treat rheumatoid arthritis and osteoarthritis. Frequently, these patients are not taken seriously, and they are told, "It is all in your head." My personal opinion is that NONRAS is a syndrome in which patients have an incomplete manifestation of the symptoms because they have a gene with the predisposition to develop this disorder. This is what I call, "muffled or buffered gene." There is no full-blown clinical manifestations of the disorder, but the gene is harmful enough to cause incapacitating joint pain more severe than osteoarthritis but not as severe as in rheumatoid arthritis. Possibly, with more research, these patients will be recognized and treated accordingly.

People commonly speak of arthritis as if it was only one type of joint disease. Typically, people refer to "arthritis" when they refer to the most common cause of joint pain: osteoarthritis (OA). However, different medical terms have their own significance such as osteoarthritis, osteoarthrosis, osteoporosis, rheumatism, chondrocalcinosis, osteopenia, osteitis, rheumatoid arthritis, and so forth.

"Arthritis" can be related to infection, connective tissue disease, hereditary types, and other entities. Physicians refer to patients using the term "arthritis" of the spine to try to explain in lay terms spinal conditions that basically mean deterioration or degeneration of the spine (spondylosis, spondylolysis, and degenerative disc disease). I suggest reading the appropriate sources of information to learn more about the above conditions.

Patients with LBP related to arthritis usually have pain in other joints in the body (shoulders, hips, hands, and so forth); however, there are certain types of "arthritis" that affect only the lower back, or they at least affect the lower back years before the affect other joints in the body.

LBP associated with arthritis typically appears as morning stiffness or pain in the lower back (and sometimes in the hands). This is pain or stiffness after being in one position for prolonged time such as sitting or lying down. The pain in the lower back is regional rather than localized or radiating (to the legs). Although, if there are spurs pressing nerves, the pain might radiate down the legs.

Pain in the joints in the lower back can cause pain radiating down the legs. Patients do not necessitate back surgery only because there is pain radiating down the legs or because there is arthritis. Not all patients with "arthritis" require surgery. A spine surgeon will decide whether surgery is warranted on "arthritis patients." Gout is a form of "arthritis" and can cause severe joint pain (and swelling).

Fibromyalgia (FM). Fibromyalgia was first described in 1904 as fibrositis. It was not until recent years that the American College of Rheumatology (ACR) coined the term fibromyalgia. Fibromyalgia can be categorized as regional, primary, secondary, and concomitant. Patients with rheumatoid arthritis, thyroid disease, and other conditions sometimes also have symptoms of fibromyalgia. We call this condition concomitant fibromyalgia.

Primary fibromyalgia is characterized by generalized musculoskeletal aching and stiffness. Researchers believe several of the above syndromes are associated and they present in combination. Others consider variants of fibromyalgia; others consider that fibromyalgia starts as one of the other syndromes.

Psychiatrists and health care providers in the area of mental care consider that fibromyalgia starts as a depressive pathology and subsequently develops into different syndromes such as fibromyalgia, chronic fatigue syndrome, myofascial pain, multiple chemical syndrome (MCS) or multiple environmental chemical syndrome, and so forth. Many of these syndromes are associated with depression, anxiety, somatization, hypochondrias, bipolar disease, personality disorders, conversion disorders, pain disorders, posttraumatic syndrome (PTS), and other somatoform disorders.

My personal opinion is that many patients with fibromyalgia and other similar syndromes have some kind of underlying depressive or personality disorder related to feelings of anguish, guilt, low self-esteem, history of child abuse, and other child trauma. Patients tend to have a feeling of self-punishment (masochism). Hormones and neurotransmitters play a role in the development of these syndromes. The biological clock claims its toll at certain ages. Genetic predisposition, along with age-related hormonal and neurotransmitter imbalances with environmental factors (including psychological changes in middle age and crisis), all make the perfect concoction for the formation of these syndromes. Depending on these factors, a body part will be affected more than other areas. Diffuse or generalized anxiety, for instance, may cause generalized symptoms such as in fibromyalgia. Psychological problems related to accepting and eliminating certain situations may cause irritable bowel syndrome (IBS) or eating disorders. Somatizations and phobias can be related to the imbalance of the above factors.

There is no clinical or scientific data to establish that trauma (physical) causes fibromyalgia. Fibromyalgia is a form of nonarticular rheumatism. The difference between fibromyalgia and other forms of musculoskeletal conditions lays in the variety, distribution, and predominance of symptoms.

How is fibromyalgia diagnosed? The diagnosis is made by excluding other organic conditions such as diabetes, thyroid disease, rheumatoid arthritis, lupus, multiple sclerosis, and so forth. Fibromyalgia is typically characterized by:

- Tender points (11 out of 18)
- Headaches
- Changes in sleeping pattern or excessive sleeping or other sleep disturbances
- Joint pain and subjective swelling
- Muscular aching and stiffness
- Weakness and fatigue
- Sensitivity to cold
- Back pain and stiffness
- Sciatica-type pain
- Chest pain
- Numbness in the limbs
- Decreased libido
- Dyspareunia (painful intercourse)
- Mood swings

- Body temperature changes from cold to hot or warm feeling
- Anxiety
- Depression
- Concentration and memory problems
- Eating disorders
- Other disturbances

FM is more frequent in females than males.

Several studies are included in the exclusion diagnosis, such as:

- Blood tests
- X-rays
- CT or MRI scan
- Endocrinologic (hormonal)
- Muscle and nerve studies
- Sleep studies
- Skin biopsy
- Psychiatric evaluation

I would need to write several pages (and possibly a book) related to this syndrome that some people call a disease. Extensive literature related to fibromyalgia can be found in different sources.

Myofascial Pain Syndrome (MPS). This is a more regional pain that is accompanied by "trigger points." It is a more benign form of fibromyalgia. It is characterized by muscle pain, and, upon pressure of the painful areas, there is a reflecting or radiating pain to another region.

Chronic Fatigue Syndrome (CFS). Mostly, fatigue, headaches, muscle aches, tender lymph nodes, sore throat, and difficulty concentrating characterize this syndrome. However, in CFS, there may be joint aches, allergies, weight loss, abdominal pain or cramps, fever, sleep disorders, and psychiatric problems.

Depression. Depression is a condition that can present with different manifestations. Depression can hide, confuse, and sometimes overlap with other conditions. It can progress in severity; it can stay dormant for several years or recur. There is a need for psychiatric evaluation to make the diagnosis, and there is a need to rule out organic conditions (labs, radiological studies, and so forth). There are several forms of depression, and the treatments vary. Depression can manifest with different symptoms such as fatigue, headaches, generalized pains, sexual dysfunction, memory problems, sleep and eating disorders, etc. Depression can be associated with other overlapping mental conditions, such as maniac/depressive personalities and neurosis. Some psychotic conditions can be characterized by depression.

Irritable Bowel Syndrome (IBS). This syndrome is characterized by abdominal pain and disturbances in bowel habits. The symptoms usually begin in late teens to early twenties.

Reflex Sympathetic Syndrome (RSD). Also known as Complex Regional Pain Syndrome type I (CRPS), it is a poorly understood syndrome in which the autonomic nerves (sympathetic) are affected and cause severe extremity pain, swelling, numbness, sometimes atrophy (muscle-wasting), and changes in skin color and temperature. Typically, there is no weakness; however, the pain can cause some degree of weakness or loss of power. Several events can cause this syndrome, such as trauma, surgery, crush injuries, injuries by sharp instruments, burns, chronic infections, diabetes, and so forth. The diagnosis of RSD is sometimes difficult to make, and it is sometimes confused with other entities. There are theories related to the cause of RSD. Causalgia is a condition that results from nerve injury and generally sharp injury. After a nerve sharp injury, there is sometimes severe extremity or limb pain called causalgia or Complex Regional Pain Syndrome II.

The treatment in either CRPS I or II is difficult. Many times, the treatment has to be done fairly soon after the diagnosis is made or suspected because the best results and outcomes have been seen on people who were treated within the first six months of the presentation of the symptoms. Typically, RSD is treated in a different way than sciatica. The treatment may involve sympathetic blocks and medications. Physical therapy (ice or heat) and surgery may sometimes aggravate the pain.

Multiple Chemical Symptoms (MCS)/Idiopathic Environmental Intolerance (IEI). This is an entity that also has psychological roots. This condition has different names, such as immune system deregulation, multiple chemical hypersensitivity, total allergy syndrome, toxic carpet syndrome and toxic response syndrome. Depression and anxiety are the core of this special condition. These conditions have been recognized since the late 1950s. Typically, an individual reports several symptoms related to exposure to chemicals and materials, such as carpets, fumes, vapors, pesticides, detergents, perfumes, and even dental amalgam. The symptoms are intertwined with those of the conditions I already mentioned, such as chronic fatigue syndrome, fibromyalgia, myofascial pain, and so forth.

In some instances, trauma (accidents such as work-related injuries, motor vehicle accidents, falls, and so forth) "triggers" some of the above conditions. The typical case would be the patient with a whiplash injury (neck pain). The patient was subconsciously waiting for a reason to start having the symptoms that otherwise would have eventually manifested with a triggering event.

Do not confuse the depression related to objective conditions related to trauma, for instance, the patient who had a severe accident and lost a leg. That patient may fall into a depressive state, and the depression may lead to a florid clinical picture with a myriad of symptoms, typical of the patient with depression. Whiplash injury generally is described for neck trauma. Whiplash injury is a well-recognized medical entity that requires treatment, and it is not "mental." However, some patients develop chronic pain or other somatoform entities after this injury.

Restless Leg Syndrome (RLS). This is an entity not necessarily related to leg pain, but some patients describe a feeling of discomfort in the legs. Some of the causes of RLS can include diabetes (peripheral neuropathy), vitamin deficiencies, intoxications, and other unusual neurological disorders.

Osteoporosis. "Osteo" refers to bone, and "porosis" refers to porous. (Thus, osteoporosis refers to "porous bone.") The bone loses minerals that cause them to become brittle and easy to break. The main mineral in the bones is calcium. But there are other minerals and vitamins important for the health of the bones. More than a million people sustained bone fractures due to osteoporosis every year. Risk factors associated with osteoporosis are low calcium intake, smoking, drinks with caffeine and high in phosphates, steroids (cortisone), chronic stress, alcohol, hormonal imbalances, low vitamin D and sun exposure, inactivity, and prolonged bed rest (bedridden patients). X-rays do not show signs of osteoporosis until about thirty percent of the bone (calcium) is disappeared.

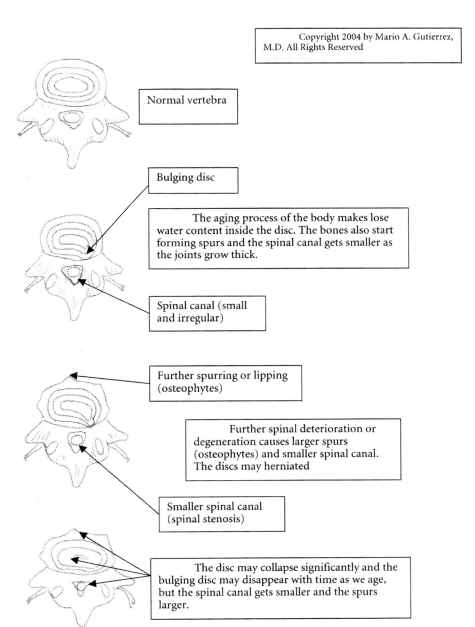

Normal vertebra

Bulging disc

The aging process of the body makes lose water content inside the disc. The bones also start forming spurs and the spinal canal gets smaller as the joints grow thick.

Spinal canal (small and irregular)

Further spurring or lipping (osteophytes)

Further spinal deterioration or degeneration causes larger spurs (osteophytes) and smaller spinal canal. The discs may herniated

Smaller spinal canal (spinal stenosis)

The disc may collapse significantly and the bulging disc may disappear with time as we age, but the spinal canal gets smaller and the spurs larger.

Stages of the spinal degenerative process.

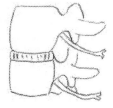

Normal spine. Lateral view (side view)

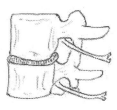

As the spine deteriorates the disc becomes smaller and it starts bulging out.

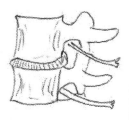

With further deterioration of the spine, the disc becomes even smaller and it protrudes more. The bones become brittle, and they tend to grow spurs on the edges. The flat surfaces of the vertebrae become curve as they lose minerals.

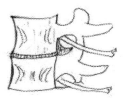

Further deterioration of the spine causes the disc (and the bones) to collapse more ("bone against bone"), the foramen get smaller, the spurs larger and the vertebral bodies become curve. People start losing height.

Side (lateral) view of the spine and stages during the degenerative or aging process.

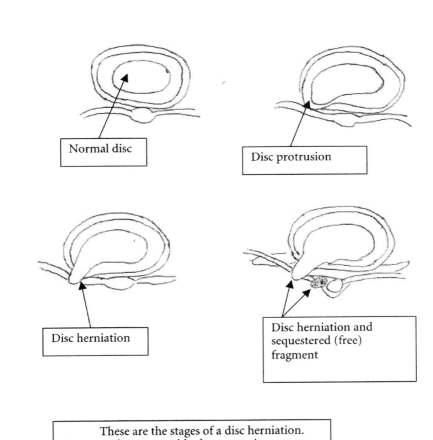

Normal disc

Disc protrusion

Disc herniation

Disc herniation and sequestered (free) fragment

These are the stages of a disc herniation. However, discs can suddenly rupture in an accident.

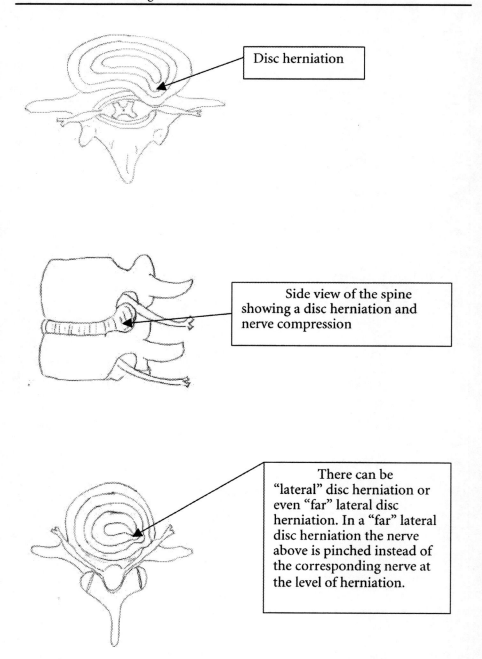

Disc herniation

Side view of the spine
showing a disc herniation and
nerve compression

There can be
"lateral" disc herniation or
even "far" lateral disc
herniation. In a "far" lateral
disc herniation the nerve
above is pinched instead of
the corresponding nerve at
the level of herniation.

Drawings representing axial views of the spine showing disc herniation
with nerve compression.

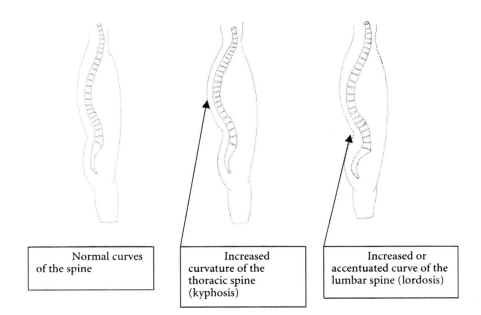

| Normal curves of the spine | Increased curvature of the thoracic spine (kyphosis) | Increased or accentuated curve of the lumbar spine (lordosis) |

Normally, there are slight curves in the spine on the lateral view. The cervical spine has a normal forward curve (lordosis), the thoracic spine has a slight backwards curve (kyphosis), and the lumbar spine has a slight forward curve (lordosis). However, exaggeration of the curves will cause abnormal deformities of the spine called kyphosis and lordosis if there is an increase in the curves of the spine. Straightening of the curves is also abnormal. Straightening in the cervical spine is called "reverse lordosis," and, if there is an increased backward deviation of the neck, it can become true kyphosis in the cervical spine. In the thoracic spine, kyphosis is more common due to collapsing of the vertebrae, such as in osteoporosis. Kyphosis is what some people call "hunchback" or "humpback." Large breasts in women can cause kyphosis. Increased lordosis in the lumbar spine can be congenital, but it can also be caused by spondylolysis and spondylolisthesis.

During the physical exam, it is important to examine the spine from the front, the back, and the side.

There can be also deviation of the spine sideways (on a front view). This is called scoliosis, and the spine may be rotated on its axis. This condition is called "rotoscoliosis." Scoliosis is usually a congenital condition, but there can also be scoliosis related to degenerative changes of the spine. Scoliosis is not always corrected because surgery sometimes increases pain. Painstaking evaluation of these patients is the norm when surgery is contemplated.

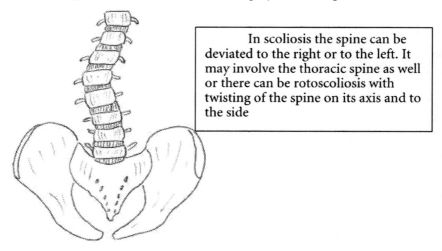

In scoliosis the spine can be deviated to the right or to the left. It may involve the thoracic spine as well or there can be rotoscoliosis with twisting of the spine on its axis and to the side

Spinal deformities throw off the balance of the spine and the gait. People tend to walk sideways or use a posture that, in time, can cause a chronic strain and sprain of the back muscles and hips. Limping or walking with an abnormal posture can cause a sacroiliac (SI) joint dysfunction that leads to LBP, hip pain, and leg pain. Amputees (with or without a prosthesis) also tend to develop SI joint dysfunction and pain.

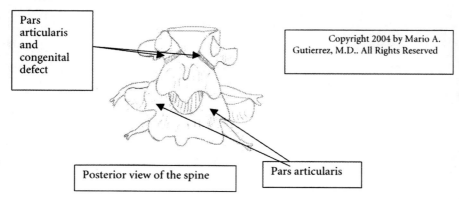

Pars articularis and congenital defect

Posterior view of the spine

Pars articularis

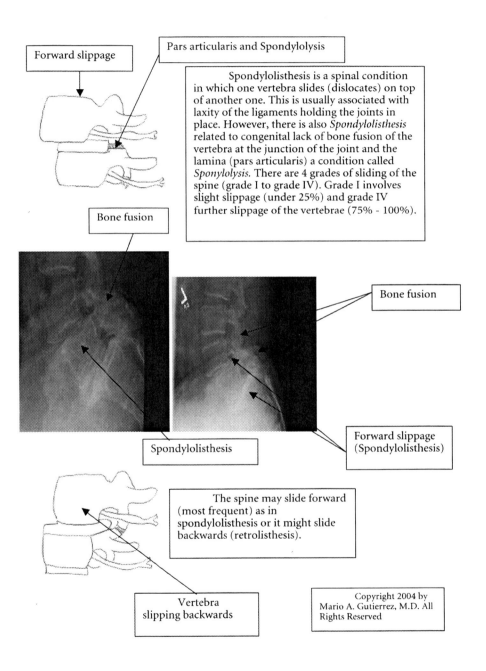

Forward slippage

Pars articularis and Spondylolysis

Spondylolisthesis is a spinal condition in which one vertebra slides (dislocates) on top of another one. This is usually associated with laxity of the ligaments holding the joints in place. However, there is also *Spondylolisthesis* related to congenital lack of bone fusion of the vertebra at the junction of the joint and the lamina (pars articularis) a condition called *Sponylolysis.* There are 4 grades of sliding of the spine (grade I to grade IV). Grade I involves slight slippage (under 25%) and grade IV further slippage of the vertebrae (75% - 100%).

Bone fusion

Bone fusion

Spondylolisthesis

Forward slippage (Spondylolisthesis)

The spine may slide forward (most frequent) as in spondylolisthesis or it might slide backwards (retrolisthesis).

Vertebra slipping backwards

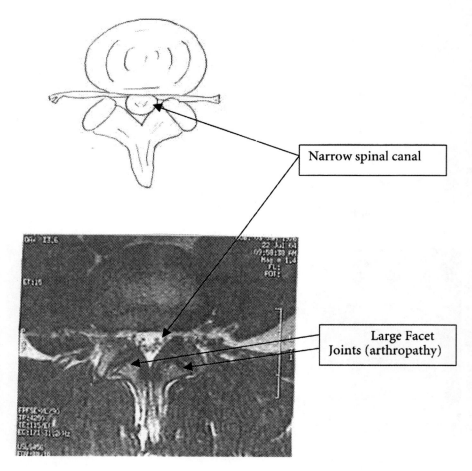

Narrow spinal canal

Large Facet
Joints (arthropathy)

Spinal stenosis or narrowing of the spinal is a common spinal condition on the aging patient.

CHAPTER 3

LBP and Diagnostic Studies

There are questions patients ask me related to studies (medical workup) necessary to diagnose LBP (and/or leg pain):

- What kind of tests do I need to have to diagnose my lower back condition?
- What are the most current tests and studies for the diagnosis of lower back conditions?
- What do the studies consist of? How are they done?
- What will they show?
- How accurate are the tests?
- Who should order the tests? Should it be the primary physician or the specialist?

Here are some of the most frequent studies used to find and diagnose causes of lower back conditions:

- Regular X-rays
- X-ray in flexion and extension (F/E) of the spine
- CAT (computerized axial tomography) scan or CT scan with and without contrast (IV dye) or with a combination of a myelogram or myelography. Helicoidal CT scan.
- MRI (magnetic resonance imaging) scan with and without contrast (IV dye)
- Bone or spinal tomogram
- EMG (electromyography)/NCV (nerve conduction velocity) studies
- Discography or discogram
- Bone scan
- Myelography

- Venography and angiography
- Bone densitometry (osteoporosis)
- Blood tests for the person with LBP and joint disease
- Somatosensory Evoked Potentials (SEPs) and Motor Evoked Responses (MEPs)
- SPECT (Single Positron Emission Computed Tomography)
- Thermotherapy (for diagnosis and treatment)
- Pain provocation and relief (facet block, epidural block, trigger point injections, nerve block, and so forth)
- Psychological tests

Some medical schools and spine centers have even designed a "cookbook" or a flowchart to follow as guidance for the diagnosis and treatment of patients with LBP. These "flowcharts" are a good guide and are acceptable; however, these flowcharts have to be used on an individual basis depending on the patient's symptoms and signs, combined with common sense and basic medical knowledge. When using flowcharts or algorithms for LBP, they generally apply only to the patient with LBP and not to the patient on an individual basis. What is important when evaluating a patient with LBP is the way of interpreting medical data, the way of collecting medical information, and the interpretation of statistical data (EBM).

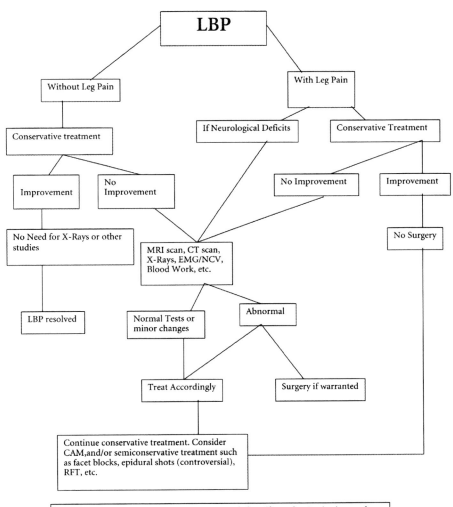

I created this simple flow chart. There are several Flow Charts that Institutions and Spine Centers have created; but one must tailor treatments to every patient.

Studies Considered Standard for the Diagnosis of a Patient with LBP

Regular or Conventional X-rays. X-rays are usually done at a hospital or physician's office. A technician takes the X-rays and most radiological studies. It does not take much time for the actual X-ray, perhaps ten to twenty minutes or less to take the X-ray and develop the film. Each test has its advantages and disadvantages; each has its own particular value for certain medical conditions. X-rays involve minimal radiation, but certain other studies may require more radiation. The X-ray involves a minimal amount of radiation when compared to a CT scan or other radiological studies. Radiation exposure should be considered when dealing with small children who are exposed to an excessive amount of radiological tests. Patients occasionally tell me they were told they have a "slipped disc" that was discovered on a regular X-ray. A regular X-ray may be of less value if the physician is looking for soft tissue injuries. Although there can be indirect signs of muscle spasm (straightening of the spine), a herniated disc will not appear on an X-ray unless the disc is calcified (that is, filled with calcium). There may be indirect findings of muscle spasm and other signs on a regular X-ray on a patient with LBP and a herniated disc. One of the most frequent tests ordered for someone with LBP is a regular X-ray. The X-ray is an excellent screening tool for bone and joint abnormalities, such as trauma, fractures, and dislocations. Cancer and bone destructive lesions also show abnormalities on regular X-rays. One can see shadows of the soft tissues and deformities of the spine (scoliosis, straightening, and so forth) on X-rays. The value of an X-ray is relative, depending on the possible causes of LBP. An X-ray may be useful when there is a history of trauma or when bone birth defects are suspected. They can be useful when cancer is suspected or when there is LBP (with or without leg pain) that lasts more than a month.

X-rays can be helpful diagnostic tools when evaluating spinal stability. They can help detect osteoporosis and compression fractures. They may be necessary before surgery to evaluate spinal stability and see the anatomy of bones. (There can be bone variants not clearly seen on an MRI scan). Otherwise, regular X-rays may not be very helpful in making a diagnosis on a patient at the beginning of an episode of LBP. Lateral X-rays can be taken on neutral, flexion, and extension of the spine while standing and lying down. (The patient is asked to bend back and forth as well as to the sides for the X-rays.) Anterior-posterior X-rays are taken on lateral flexion of the spine to check for stability. For someone who bent over and twisted the lower back ("a pulled muscle"), chances are that we will see only indirect evidence of muscle spasm on the X-rays. If there is a herniated disc, X-rays will not show it. Therefore, X-rays may

not be very useful in some patients with LBP. The legal system has great influence in the medical decision-making process when ordering X-rays on a
patient with LBP. Physicians order X-rays even though they know X-rays will
not show a herniated disc and other spinal conditions, but they order them to
satisfy the patient. (Many times, patients request X-rays.) Other times, physicians also order X-rays to satisfy medical institutions or the medical community. Recent studies focus on the necessity and use of conventional X-rays for
the patient with LBP. The results of the studies are (as we would expect) as follows: There is increased expense in unnecessary X-rays in most patients.
However, a positive psychological impact has been noticed in patients who felt
"comfortable" with what the physician is doing to help. A positive effect on the
patient's recovery and treatment has been observed when the patient had X-
rays taken. Patients think the physician is "doing something." This has more
psychological value than physical.

I would not recommend X-rays on a young person with LBP if the mechanism of injury was trivial and if I suspect a sprain/strain. For a patient with a
history of a fall, car accident, trauma, or suspected cancer, I would definitively
recommend X-rays. I usually order regular X-rays on older people with LBP
because the chances of cancer or arthritis are more likely than in younger
patients. Depending on the type of pain and other factors (obtained from the
medical history and physical), I may order X-rays. If the patient has chronic
LBP and leg pain with worsening of the pain, an MRI scan could be indicated
as the first study. For a patient who already had low back surgery, an MRI scan
with and without contrast (IV dye) would be indicated before any other test if
there is a suspected recurrence of an injury or new injuries. What is the best
first test that should be done on a patient with LBP: a thorough medical history and physical exam. When the physician has obtained a medical history
and when a physical exam has been performed, what is the next step to make
diagnosis? The decision for more tests is directly related to the medical history
and the physical exam. Sometimes, there is no need to run any test at all. The
first test we order depends on where we suspect the pain is most likely originating. Several tests are available to the physician to diagnose a patient with
LBP. There are instances or cases in which the cause of LBP or leg pain cannot
be pinpointed with certainty. There is another type of X-ray called tomogram
or tomography. A computerized X-ray machine takes slices of sections of body
parts. This study shows only the bones.

**CT (Computerized Tomography)/CAT (Computerized Axial Tomography)
Scan.** This is a radiological study in which slices of body parts are taken. The
difference between an X-ray and a CT scan is that soft tissues are viewed on a
CT scan. The CT (CAT) scan machine is the predecessor of the MRI scan. One

can order a CT scan of the spine, the abdomen, the sacrum bone, or different body parts. The CT scan can be obtained with and without IV contrast (dye) to better define the anatomy of the body part scanned. The patient must notify the physician and the CT scan technician if there is a history of allergic reactions to IV dye so that the dye will not be used. A CT scan can be done after injecting dye into the spine (subarachnoid space). This study is called myelogram/CT scan. This study enhances the anatomy of the spinal cord and nerves. A technician usually performs this test at a hospital. It may take about fifteen to thirty minutes plus another fifteen minutes to develop the film. If there is a need for preparation for the study, it may take longer depending on the generation and the brand of the machine, as some machines are faster than others.

The patient should remain still while undergoing the CT scan to get a good quality study (as with MRI scan studies). CT scan is a test that had a great deal of importance when it first came into the medical field several years ago. This test also involves radiation and is an excellent tool not only for bony structures but also for screening soft tissues. However, a CT scan is outdated in some instances compared to an MRI scan. The CT scan can be an excellent complementary radiodiagnostic tool to the MRI scan.

The main application of a spinal CT scan is for diagnosing spinal stenosis, spinal trauma, herniated nucleus pulposus, spinal tumor (bone tumor mainly), and for patients with LBP after surgery. However, the CT scan has some other indirect applications. The advantage of the CT scan is that it takes minimal time for the study and is done in an open machine (opposed to an MRI scan that is done in an enclosed machine). (Some patients are claustrophobic.) CT scans are also less expensive than MRI scans. The CT scan gives excellent pictures of the bones and soft tissues. However, the CT scan had some limitations until a new version was invented: a helicoidal CT scan that gives a 3-D (three-dimensional) picture. The old CT scan is still used at most medical facilities and is only 2-D (two-dimensional). With a CT scan, transversal (across) and vertical slices of the body are viewed. The CT scan of the lumbar spine has some limitations for soft tissues when compared to an MRI scan. A CT scan is excellent for bone [fracture, dislocation or subluxation, spurs (osteophytes), and deformities] but not for the subtle soft tissue changes (as MRI scan is). There are certain rural areas in which an MRI scan machine is unavailable. Under these circumstances, the CT scan is a good screening tool and is a good neurodiagnostic tool for the evaluation of a patient with LBP. There are CT machines of excellent resolution (picture definition) in which the image is so clear that it is rare to also require an MRI scan if the CT scan shows no obvious abnormalities. Response to medical treatment will also dictate what tests to order on a patient with LBP.

MRI (Magnetic Resonance Imaging) Scan. An MRI is the gold standard for diagnosis on patients with spinal conditions. This study is usually performed at a hospital or in a mobile unit. A technician does the study; a radiologist interprets the films. The MRI scan machine is often an enclosed "tube" into which the patient is taken while lying on a mobile table. There are special units that are open, and there are special units for large people. The MRI machine frequently supports patients that weigh up to 236 pounds, but there are patients with a wide chest and abdomen that do not fit into the machine. It may take from twenty to thirty-five minutes for the study or longer if there are motion artifacts on the films (if the patient moves while having the study done). It takes another ten to fifteen minutes to develop the films. During the test, a technician is giving instructions to the patient through an intercom from inside a small room. The MRI scan may be obtained with an IV dye (contrast) to enhance the anatomy of the spine. The patient should always notify the physicians and the MRI scan technician if he or she has claustrophobia or if the patient has any metal in the body. Some patients who experience claustrophobia may require sedation. To obtain an MRI scan, an MRI technician routinely should ask the patient about metal in the body. It is dangerous to do an MRI scan on a patient with a pacemaker. The machine acts as a large magnet that could pull metallic objects from inside the body or it can cause motion or dislodgment of aneurysm clips and so forth. The patient should always notify the physicians and the technician at the time of the MRI scan if there is any metal in the body (prosthesis, pacemaker, programmable VP shunt, etc).

The MRI scan involves magnetic fields, not involve radiation. Through a computerized system using magnetic fields, it reads the biological composition (water) of the tissues and sends an image back to the computer, which the machine interprets. So far, no adverse effects over the body have been reported with MRI scans. Its effects on health have not clearly been defined. The MRI scan is the Cadillac of the tests for the brain, spine, and other body organs. It has some limitations and should be included in the workup along with other tests, such as conventional X-rays, CT scans, myelograms, discograms, and so forth. By itself, an MRI scan may be sufficient to make a diagnosis and to recommend surgery. The MRI scan may show definitive, clear-cut information so that no other tests will be required for treatment. In some instances, other tests may add certain information to MRI scan findings. Some orthopedic surgeons and neurosurgeons may want to get more tests when a spinal fusion procedure is considered. When spinal instability is suspected, regular X-rays have an invaluable role (flexion-extension views of the spine). Although the MRI scan provides excellent views of the spine, it does not test the spine for stability. In this case, the MRI scan has its limitation.

Myelogram or Myelography. This is a study usually done by a physician (radiologist, orthopedic surgeon, or neurosurgeon) at a hospital; a short outpatient stay is often required. It may take from twenty to forty-five minutes, depending on the difficulty encountered when placing the needle into the spine. This is one of the oldest tests done for neurodiagnostic purposes. This test was used many years ago when neither MRI nor CT scan studies were available. Different dyes have been used throughout the years. The more current dyes are less toxic. Current dyes are absorbed into the spinal fluid. In the old times, the dye was oily and it had to be removed after the injection for a myelogram. Even today, side effects may occur due to allergic or chemical reactions to the dye. Radiation is involved in this study. (Typically, it is more radiation than one receives for a regular X-ray). It is a procedure that involves a spinal tap. The patient should notify the physician if he or she has allergies to local anesthetic medications, dyes, or chemicals. If the patient had the same study done before, the patient must notify the physician if there were complications, such as headaches, nausea, vomiting, or other adverse reactions.

It is extremely important to notify the physician if the patient is on blood thinners at the time of the study. This study cannot be done under these circumstances because a spinal hemorrhage may occur. A hemorrhage can lead to serious spinal cord damage and paralysis. Some blood thinners are the following: aspirin, anti-inflammatory medications, Coumadin, Plavix, Heparin, Lovenox, TPA, Aggrenox, Persantine, and other medications used for stroke, heart attack, pulmonary embolism, and deep venous thrombosis (DVT). It is important for the physicians to know if the patient has leukemia, hemophilia, or some other coagulation disorder. Some antibiotics such as Keflex (cephalosporin) can be associated with an increased chance for hemorrhage.

To perform a myelogram, local anesthesia is injected into the skin. Then a long needle is inserted through the spine into the area of the nerves. Usually, spinal fluid will come out. It will be collected for specific laboratory studies. A dye is injected into the subarachnoid space to define more precisely the spinal cord and the nerves in the X-rays. X-rays are taken after the dye has been injected. The patient is to remain still while the dye is being injected into the subarachnoid space (into the spinal fluid) to avoid damaging the nerves. The radiologist may ask the technician to change the table to different positions (that is, tilting the table) to move the dye to the area the physician is interested in evaluating.

Complications from the spinal tap may include headaches, nausea and vomiting, spinal or brain hemorrhage, nerve damage, scar tissue and arachnoiditis, spinal fluid leak, and other complications. It is important to immediately notify the physician who did the test and the primary care physician if the patient develops numbness, tingling or weakness in the legs, or difficulty urinating or with bowel control following the test. Some of these symptoms could be related to a spinal hemorrhage or infection that will require emergency radiological studies and possibly surgery. Late complications may occur such as infection and scar tissue (arachnoiditis) with resulting increased LBP. Arachnoiditis is less frequent with the use of current dyes opposed to the nonsoluble dyes used several years ago. Arachnoiditis is inflammation of the arachnoid membrane. (Refer to the glossary for more information.)

Some surgeons use myelogram plus flexion and extension films and a CT scan of the lumbar spine for evaluation when a spinal fusion with hardware is being considered. Sometimes, it is difficult to assess the lateral recess (refer to spinal anatomy) with only an MRI scan. The myelogram/CT scan may add additional information to an MRI scan and is valuable when considering a surgical approach, for example, an intra- or extraforaminal decompression.

After a myelogram has been performed, the patient has to remain flat in bed approximately six to eight hours to decrease the chances of complications, such as headaches, nausea, and vomiting due to loss of spinal fluid. A spinal tap can be fatal on someone who has an undiscovered brain lesion or a tumor. After a spinal tap, a patient can die from herniation of the brain through the foramen magnum, which is the hole at the base of the skull through which the brain stem joins the spinal cord. With negative pressure exerted by the spinal tap and CSF leak, the brain stem is sucked down into the upper area of the spinal cord, collapsing the vital functions of the brain. This complication is rare; however, the physician must get a good medical history and exam that will provide clues to suspect brain tumor before doing this study. With the arrival of the MRI scan, fewer physicians are using invasive procedures such as myelograms. Some physicians do only the spinal tap, the injection of the dye, and the CT scan without the actual myelogram (regular X-rays of the spine while the dye is in the subarachnoid space).

Discogram or Discography. A radiologist or an orthopedic surgeon typically does this study at a hospital. It is an injection of dye into the disc itself, and X-rays are taken after the injection. Some physicians consider this test to be of double diagnostic value. If the patient experiences leg pain during the procedure, it is suspected the disc itself is degenerated and the disc is the cause of LBP and leg pain. The other value of the test is to check the shape of the disc. The disc may be out of place. Currently, there is controversy about this study among physicians, orthopedic surgeons, neurosurgeons, and other clinicians who deal with patients with LBP. Some physicians claim that, if an MRI scan does not show a herniated disc, the discogram will not show any more information. In some institutions, physicians have used the term internal derangement or internal disc herniation for certain cases. They claim internal disc herniation can be better viewed in a discogram. The value of this study is to be taken with caution. The interpretation of a discogram can be based on personal experience. There can be complications from this study, such as nerve damage, spinal fluid leak, increased pain, or infection (discitis and bone infection). Recently, studies have described cases of disc herniation caused by the study. Studies of a discogram and MRI scan together are still in the experimental phase.

EMG (Electromyography)/NCV (Nerve Conduction Velocity) Studies. These studies are done typically at a hospital or physician's office. Physicians perform the EMG, but a technician does the NCV. The electromyography has its unique value. Needles are applied into the muscle of a limb or the trunk, and electrical stimulation is applied to measure the response of the muscle. The placement of the needle into the muscles is usually painful. Of course, the needles should be sterile.

As part of the NCV study, the nerves are tested with another device applied directly onto the skin over a nerve. Electrical stimulation is applied. The nerve response is recorded. These two studies (EMG/NCV) are of excellent value for muscular and nerve disorders. They also provide excellent information about the age of the disorder and whether there is an acute or a chronic nerve condition. When compared with previous EMG/NCV studies, they are of diagnostic and prognostic value. It takes about sixty minutes to perform the studies.

Single Positron Emission Computed Tomography Scanning (SPECT or PET Scan). This is a study that is particularly useful for patients with some degree of spinal instability, and it detects patients with spondylolysis. It is also useful for patients with postoperative pain when instability is suspected (pars articularis defect). Pseudoarthrosis can be detected with a SPECT when bone fusion surgery took place.

Muscular and/or Nerve Biopsy. A physician typically performs these studies at a hospital or in his or her office. These unusual studies are done when systemic disorders such as multiple sclerosis (MS), amyotrophic lateral sclerosis (ALS), muscular dystrophy, or other disorders are suspected. The specimen must be taken to a pathology laboratory. These biopsies are performed using a local anesthetic. They may take from ten to twenty minutes. More time may be required if performing a nerve biopsy. The patient has to notify the physicians about allergies to medications or anesthetics. There is risk of complications such as nerve damage, pain (temporary or permanent), infection, and hemorrhage.

Somatosensory Evoked Potential Studies (SSEPs)/Motor Evoked Potentials Studies (MEPs). These tests are primarily done for the upper part of the spine at the cervical or thoracic regions or in the area of the brain stem. They are rarely used during the LBP workup. However, they are sometimes used during spinal surgery.

Bone Scan. A bone scan is a study in which a radionuclide IV dye specific for bone is used. In this study, the skeleton is seen on a picture. Certain disorders can be diagnosed with this study. In suspected bone cancer or metastasis, a bone scan study is the gold standard. Fractures and other bone conditions can also be diagnosed with a bone scan. Sometimes, the negativity of certain tests are of diagnostic value (by ruling out disorders), such as in myeloma multiple (bone destructive lesion). In some cases, X-rays show bone destructive lesions, but the bone scan could be normal.

Bone Density Test. This test is done primarily on people in which osteoporosis is suspected. This test measures the density of the bones (that is, the amount of calcium).

There are *other studies* that are focused to detect specific unusual disorders, for instance, the Tensilon test for myasthenia gravis.

Special laboratory tests are done for specific diseases. Blood, urine, CSF, or other biological fluids are studied for specific disorders, such as infestation for parasites, chronic infections, Lyme disease, rickettsiosis, and so forth. Blood work is necessary when certain bone and joint conditions are suspected (for example, rheumatoid arthritis, lupus, multiple sclerosis, infection, cancer, and so forth). Usually, a basic preoperative set of studies and lab tests are ordered on all patients. Patients younger than thirty years old usually do not need a chest X-ray and EKG unless there is a previous medical condition that warrants these tests (for example, patients with congenital or acquired heart or lung conditions). People on dialysis or specific treatments for certain disorders will also need specific tests.

For patients over thirty years of age, I usually order a chest X-ray, EKG, urine for analysis and cultures with sensitivity, CBC, and blood chemistry. When there is a history of hemorrhagic conditions, there is a need to order bleeding time, PT, PTT, platelets, and other special bleeding tests. Some surgeons order regular X-rays of the lumbar spine before surgery in addition to other studies such as MRI scan, CT scan, bone scan, etc. Other surgeons order neutral, flexion, and extension films and even lateral flexion X-rays of the spine to test for stability. It is important to get bone density studies, especially on older patients, patients that have been on steroids, and patients prone to have osteoporosis. Bone density tests are particularly important when a spinal fusion surgery with instrumentation has been planned. (Spinal fusion with hardware may be contraindicated on patients with osteoporosis.) The weak, brittle bone may break if hardware is used.

Certain tests are important before surgery, such as pulmonary function tests (PFTs) for patients with lung disease or smokers. Liver function tests (LFTs) are important on patients with a history of liver disease. Renal (kidney) studies are necessary for patients who are to undergo spinal surgery and have a history of renal failure or insufficiency.

Patients with heart disease may need to have cardiac tests, such as EKG, a stress test, and echocardiogram. It is not recommended to do any elective major surgery on patients who had a heart attack within six months until they are stable and cleared by a cardiologist. Patients who have hemophilia, who are Jehovah's Witness, and who have certain medical conditions represent special challenges for the surgeon.

Patients with lupus or cancer represent a medical challenge because of possible complications after surgery. Surgery, as a traumatic event for the body, is also a stressful situation that could trigger major events and complications for people with certain disorders. The surgeon should be prepared to deal with potential complications and get other specialists involved in the postoperative care.

The physician should order certain tests in a prudent manner. The physician should be familiar with his or her hospital and community plus the available manpower and equipment resources. I believe it is a good approach to initially order an MRI scan of the lumbar spine if there is clinical reason to order it.

Are most tests physicians order justified? I believe they are. However, an excess of tests is done in this country. This phenomenon is due to the American legal system. Physicians practice what is called "defensive medicine," which is a way of practicing medicine by ordering excessive tests to avoid liability.

A medical workup should be tailored to the patient's age, body structure, life style, interest, medical history, and physical examination. The most likely cause of LBP dictates the workup.

No test can be a substitute for a good clinical history and exam. No test can be a substitute for the physician's judgment.

Pitfalls in the Interpretation of Radiodiagnostic Studies

In 1993, the *New England Journal of Medicine* published an article related to abnormalities found on MRI scans performed on people with no history of LBP. After this publication, there have been other studies with the same results. In general, a great percentage of people showed abnormalities on the MRI scan. These are some of the results: The prevalence of disc degeneration (degenerative disc disease or DDD) can vary from forty-six to ninety-three percent on ages fifty to sixty and over. Collapsed discs, disc herniations, protruding discs, and bulging discs have been found on these studies.

On ages twenty to fifty, disc degeneration by MRI scan was found in as much as seventy-two to ninety percent of people. Not surprisingly, the older the person, the higher incidence of disc degeneration. There is also a high prevalence of degenerative spinal changes in the younger population. Furthermore, these disc degenerative changes do not necessarily correlate clinically with the type of LBP and with the severity of the pain. New studies on lower back diagnosis and treatment provide useful medical information, but, at the same time, they create confusion in the medical and legal systems. Examples of confusing situations with diagnosis and treatment are in the workers' compensation and third-party liability settings. Diagnosing someone with DDD may have several implications.

The finding of DDD could have a psychological impact on a patient. This condition has an impact on social and financial situation. The discovery of an abnormal MRI scan may lead a person to quit a job. Litigation is always lurking in the workers' compensation, third-party, or car accident environments. An abnormal spine MRI scan can bring legal issues related to obtaining new health insurance coverage.

There are physicians who have used the term "LBP of unknown origin." This diagnosis can be confusing to some insurance companies, attorneys, and patients. Vague diagnosis may give the impression to the layperson, insurance companies, or attorneys that the "doctor does not know what he or she is doing." A patient may worry the doctor does not have a clue of what is wrong. However, it is true that, many times, a physician does not know with certainty the origin of LBP.

An abnormal MRI scan showing degenerative disc disease is not absolute proof that this is the origin of LBP. Discograms also have false positive results. If an MRI scan shows degenerative spinal changes, it is assumed the pain is related to these abnormalities. Pain generators can be facet joints, the hips, ligaments, muscles, or other structures in the lower back. One must exercise clinical judgment when making a diagnosis and when treating a patient with LBP.

Degenerative disc disease does not occur because of one single accident. The physician may expect to see fractures, dislocations, and so forth because of trauma. The degenerative processes occur over time, over several months, or over years. There are cases in which (the majority) the person never experienced LBP before being involved in a car accident, a work-related accident, or some other incident or activity (lifting, bending, and so forth). These situations may trigger symptoms on a spine that already had degenerative changes. I have seen in my practice that this is the most frequent event. I will discuss under the workers' compensation section terms such as aggravation, exacerbation, precipitation, recurrence, and acceleration. Most states follow general rules of workers' compensation in which "preexisting conditions" are recognized as degenerative conditions, but the triggering mechanism or accident causing the symptoms is still under workers' compensation coverage.

When a patient has LBP and has physical therapy or spinal adjustments and manipulations, the patient may experience more LBP or leg pain and intervertebral disc ruptures. There is the question if a disc herniation occurred because of the physical therapy and/or manipulations…or was the disc already ruptured before the treatments? Other questions can be: Was the patient prone to develop this complication from spinal manipulations? Was it necessary to obtain an MRI scan before doing physical therapy and/or manipulations and adjustments? Some of these situations become difficult to establish and handle when there is an abnormal spine MRI scan.

In general, I do not recommend overzealous manipulations and adjustments of the spine on patients over thirty years of age because of the high incidence of degenerative changes in the spine and the susceptibility for complications from these practices.

More Comments on Other Radiological Studies Including MRI Scan

Physicians advocate that "X-rays should be the exception rather than the rule" when it comes to diagnosis and treating a patient with LBP. However, this is a relative statement. There are clear indications for radiological studies, specifically for conventional X-rays. Trauma is a well-accepted indication for X-rays. In fact, X-rays are the best tools to diagnose bone conditions such as fracture, tumor, infection, subluxation (dislocation), and so forth. There is a great deal of expense—not to mention radiation exposure—involved in X-rays. Patients need to learn that X-rays are often not necessarily required when someone has LBP.

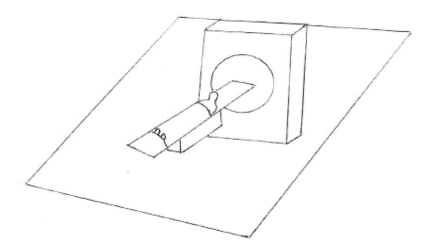

CT scan is one of the most valuable diagnostic tools for LBP.

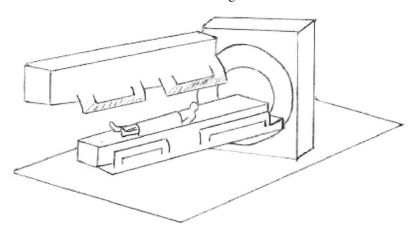

MRI scan is the "gold standard" for diagnosis of patients with LBP. Patients must notify the physician, the personnel, and the technicians if there is a history of claustrophobia so that special arrangements are made to obtain an MRI scan. There is an "open" MRI scan machine, which is much more convenient for large patients and patients with a history of claustrophobia.

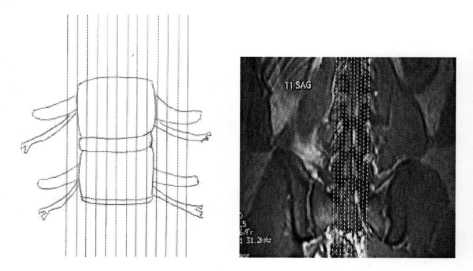

Typically, vertical (sagittal) and horizontal (axial) slices are obtained when doing an MRI scan. This drawing represents a vertical (or sagittal) slice of the spine.

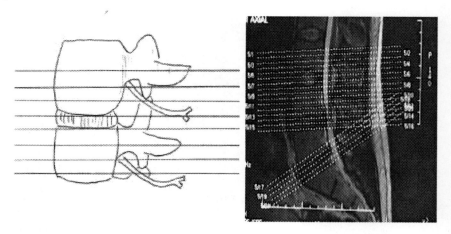

Horizontal (axial) slices of the spine are obtained during an MRI scan.

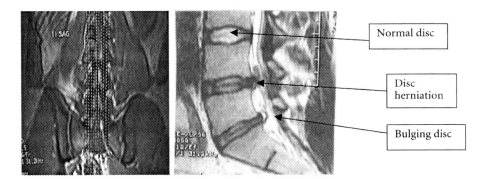

Sagittal (vertical) slices. Side (lateral) view of the spine.
(MRI scan)

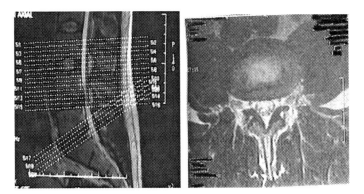

Axial (horizontal) slices of the spine. Axial (up-down) view of the spine.

On an MRI scan, one can also get coronal slices of the body (and spine). This would be a front view of the spine.

Questions

Why do I have LBP? There are different sources of back pain such as bones, discs, ligaments, tendons, and muscles. LBP can be related to internal organs and to systemic disorders. There are several causes of LBP. I have listed causes of LBP in this chapter.

The pain can be related to different conditions. These conditions can be age-related. I start going through differential diagnoses as soon as I see a patient walking into my office. However, this "first-sight diagnosis" is closely age-related. My diagnoses vary if the patient is seventeen or seventy-one years of age. On the seventeen-year-old patient, I think of a strain/sprain. On the seventy-one-year-old patient, I think of degenerative spine changes or cancer.

A visit with a primary care physician will help the patient find the cause of the pain, especially if the pain is lasting or lingering for more than one or two weeks.

Over the age of fifty, degenerative spine conditions are the leading cause of LBP. Over the age of sixty, tumor and cancer should always be suspected, particularly if the pain is severe and localized to the spine area.

Can LBP be a hereditary condition that would make me prone to develop low back problems early in life? Yes. As any other physical genetic trait and medical condition, we do have the genetic information to be strong and weak in certain organs and systems in our bodies. Therefore, there is some predisposition to have spine conditions at an early age when we have a family history of spine problems. This answer leads to another question: What can I do to avoid low back surgery if a family member already had it? The answer is to use common sense. Do not abuse the spine doing physical activities, sports, poor posture, and activities or habits (for example, smoking) that could accelerate the degenerative spine process. Avoid obesity. Stay in good physical condition and fitness. Watch the diet, and exercise on a regular basis (that is, exercises that will increase muscle strength and cardiovascular activities). Avoid exercises and activities that could deteriorate the spine or could injure it. Refer to the section in this book related to physical therapy and special low back exercises.

Is age an important factor in developing LBP? Certain age-related conditions are frequently related to LBP.

What kind of studies or tests do I need to find the cause of my LBP? The age, the history, and the physical exam will dictate the study that most likely will give information to the physician. Again, the age of presentation of the painful condition is an important factor to determine the kind of studies needed. A simple X-ray may be the first and only study we need. Perhaps a bone scan or EMGs/NCVs might be the first tests to order. Blood studies are of particular importance to rule out an underlying joint disease or another systemic disease. An abdominal X-ray, ultrasound, or some other study may be indicated to rule out an abdominal or pelvic disorder. It is up to the physician to decide which study will most likely find the source of the pain. Studies may not be authorized by health insurance companies as managed care and HMOs are having more influence in the decision-making process They may follow a cookbook, a flowchart, or some algorithm presented and recognized by a prestigious journal.

CHAPTER 4

Treatment

History of the Treatment of LBP

The treatment of LBP goes back as far as 2500 BC. In Greece, ancient physicians treated patients with LBP. Aesculap was one of the ancient physicians who used divine and human theories to treat patients. Plato referred to Aesculap as a "scientist" because, prior to him, medicine was purely a divine act. Aesculap died in 1190 BC. Hippocrates was born on the island of Kos, Greece, around 460 BC. He died in Larissa, Greece, around 377 or 390 BC. He is considered the father of scientific medicine. He also made important observations in the field of medicine and contributions to orthopedics and the treatment of patients with spinal conditions, including trauma (fractures) and degenerative diseases. The Hippocratic collection (as many as sixty books in medicine) called Corpus Hippocraticus includes his "Peri Agmon" and "Peri Arthron," as well as ancient treatments for the spine.

Galen (129–213 AD), another important ancient physician, made significant contributions to medicine (anatomy). There was a great deal of medical science knowledge in ancient cities such as Alexandria, Athens, Corinth, Syria, Macedonia, and Cyprus. These physicians described the principles of spinal anatomy and some rudimentary treatments, such as traction for patients with spinal deformities, manipulation for those with LBP and scoliosis, and other forms of treatment. For centuries, there was little treatment of patients with LBP other than nebulous techniques used by "healers," such as bed rest, manipulations, traction, and so forth. It was not until recently that many forms of treatment have been developed for patients with LBP. Currently, within the last fifty years, there has been more research and knowledge of the mechanics, anatomy, and treatment of the spine.

Currently, there are several treatment options for the patient with LBP:

- No treatment at all

- Conservative
- Semiconservative and minimally invasive procedures
- Complementary and alternative medicine (CAM)
- Surgery
- Gene therapy (still experimental)
- Radiation and chemotherapy for patients with cancer (gamma knife radiation has been tried on patients with scar tissue and failed back surgery)

Patients have the idea that we, physicians, should do all the work and cure them from any illness. If I would break down the percentage of influential factors in the treatment of a patient, I would break it down this way:

- Thirty percent of the treatment of a patient may reside in the physician's treatment.
- Thirty percent of the treatment has to do with the patient accepting responsibility and being compliant.
- Twenty percent is rehabilitation (for example, physical therapy, body posture and good body mechanics, and avoidance of activities that may endanger the treatment rendered by health care providers).
- Twenty percent of the treatment lays on Mother Nature and time to heal.

(This is an arbitrary way of explaining the multiple factors involved in the treatment of a patient.) I believe it is not wise not to treat a patient with a painful condition, particularly if serious implications may arise for not treating the patient. If the body expresses pain, it is because that body part needs attention. There are conditions that have specific guides for treatment. However, when speaking of patients with LBP, the treatment should be tailored to the patient's needs, lifestyle, and other issues discussed later in this chapter.

There are myths related to the treatment of low back conditions that I will discuss later in this book. There are also the well-known **algorithms**, flowcharts, and follow-the-instructions guides. These approaches are not necessarily wrong because they give not only medical guidelines, but also help physicians follow standards of care when legal aspects are involved in the treatment of people with low back conditions.

Different schools and medical institutions have developed some of these algorithms. These institutions take the name of "back clinic," "back institute," and others. The institutions or clinics are typically well-organized systems with several specialists working in a team. Hundreds of back surgeries are performed in these institutions and clinics every year. They follow protocols and algorithms for the treatment of a patient with LBP. I believe they would experience results that are more successful if they were to individualize treatment on a case-by-case basis.

I also want to emphasize there is a tendency to generalize the information obtained in popular magazines, journals, and even medical textbooks regarding patients with low back and leg pain. There are patients who never experience LBP, only leg pain. How do these books or magazines categorize these patients? What do they recommend for their treatment? All information and medical literature is accessible to anyone in public places like libraries, the Internet, and other computerized data banks. Everyone now has this information at his or her fingertips; however, it can be misleading. In fact, one should take the information very carefully and obtain a recommendation from a physician or specialist. Some of this information, however, can be used to ask the proper questions. Some insurance companies reject surgery automatically if conservative treatment was not attempted initially.

Currently, studies in reputable spinal publications are more realistic, and they analyze groups of people on a more individual basis. These studies also mention that the previous studies on patients with LBP may not be accurate. A patient must be cautious before making any hasty decision on certain treatments for LBP, especially if the treatment involves invasive procedures such as surgery.

When a patient has some kind of cancer, one is willing to try anything, even experimental procedures or treatments (medications, drugs, and so forth). However, we have to remember that many of these studies are only experimental, and they usually do not have enough data to know results, possible adverse outcomes, and complications. University hospitals typically perform these studies, and only they can afford from the legal standpoint these experimental treatments and surgeries. One must be cautious about these "guinea pig" studies. These treatments sometimes worsen the disease and cause patients to have more complications or even death. This is when a specialist should discuss the pros and cons of an experimental treatment.

There is no doubt that current treatments in medicine have evolved a great deal, but the basic principles of the spine remain the same. The goals of spinal surgery remain the same as in ancient times: improve the patient's condition, avoid further damage, and not cause more damage. Newer surgical techniques are innovative and ingenious, but they sometimes defy the laws of nature and physics.

More significantly, some surgical techniques overlook common sense and instinct. We have to apply the logistics of physics. A scientist, such as a physician, tends to think in a linear manner without considering variants such as the human factor, patient's lifestyle, physical and psychology structure, and so forth. If the spine is "crooked," one must straighten it out. That is a linear simplistic way of thinking when considering the human body.

There are spine surgeons who think that, if a patient with a long-standing scoliosis (sideways crooked spine) undergoes corrective surgery, the condition may actually get worse and result in more pain. The question always remains: How much is too much? Should I straighten the spine out to the one hundred percent normal anatomy? These are the kind of dilemmas that no one can answer with certainty, but one must use basic scientific knowledge, common sense, experience, and instinct based on individual basis (EBM).

One can read from different sources the general treatment for patients with LBP. The studies sometimes do not specify the cause of LBP. Even in medical textbooks in which the treatment is mentioned for someone with a specific disorder such as disc herniation or spinal stenosis, physicians only mention the general treatment. Professional medical textbooks will state the treatment should be tailored to a specific condition.

The treatment for elderly patients with LBP and several medical conditions such as heart disease, diabetes, hypertension, and lung disease differs from the otherwise young patient. We treat a patient with a condition, not a condition on a patient.

In my practice, some indicators give me an idea of the most appropriate treatment for a specific person. I consider several factors. There are situations in which there is no doubt that surgery is the solution without even attempting "conservative treatment."

Recent studies favor early surgery, contrary to what was believed not long ago. Patients have much better outcome, recovery, and productivity when surgery is done at an early stage of the condition and when a reputable, experienced surgeon recommends surgery. Studies have indicated that the longer a patient takes to get relief of the symptoms either with or without surgery, the less chances of ever going back to work. The longer the pain and symptoms linger, the more chances for a vicious cycle of pain, depression, frustration, anger, more pain, and less productivity. The longer a nerve is compressed, the more chances for nerve damage and the longer recovery may take.

Surgeons must be cautious when electing to use a specific surgical technique. There are some considerations I make when debating between the performance of a microdiskectomy and a diskectomy (or microdiskectomy) with spinal fusion (or a more aggressive surgery). The success rate of a microdiskectomy without fusion is high, varying from seventy to ninety percent, according to the studies we review. The success rate of a diskectomy with fusion varies depending on the kind of instrumentation used. (There are different companies that sell different products.) The outcome also depends on several aspects of the patient.

There is another consideration. If a microdiskectomy without fusion fails to significantly improve the patient and if the patient needs another surgery, the patient still has other options. If the patient who has a spinal instrumentation fusion fails to improve, the patient might experience more pain, and few options are left for further treatment and surgery. In order to perform a spinal fusion, bone sometimes has to be removed (parts of the joints). Removal of the joints destabilizes the spine; therefore, it is imperative that some kind of hardware is used to keep the spine stable. This is a disadvantage in spinal instrumentation. The approach should not cause more harm, pain, or neurological deficits (numbness or weakness).

Spinal instrumentation is an excellent approach when it works and when it is indicated. The question each surgeon has is: When is a spinal fusion indicated? There is controversy on the indications for fusion surgery for one disc herniation. I will discuss indications and contraindications for surgery in more detail later in this chapter.

Many spine surgeons refer their patients to "pain clinics" when their operations do not work. Sometimes, these patients with a "failed back surgery" are sent to another spine specialist for more surgery. Have you heard of those patients who had more than one surgery, are on a morphine pump, require narcotic pain medications around the clock, or are scheduled for more surgeries? Typically, these patients underwent a spinal fusion first for a noncomplicated disc herniation.

Age, previous medical conditions that may contraindicate surgery or may increase complication rate, as well as type of personality, social habits, body size, and other medical disorders are important facts to consider for election of treatment.

If a textbook says the best treatment for a specific condition is a determined surgical technique, the surgeon isolates and leaves the patient out of the decision-making process. There are only few conditions that one would consider as clear-cut indications for surgery, such as severe LBP associated with leg pain and neurological symptoms of numbness, weakness, and sphincter dysfunction. These can be indications for emergency or elective surgery. The majority of patients remain in a great gray area. Different surgical techniques could be applied to a large population of patients with LBP.

Surgical techniques should be tailored not only to the patient's condition but also to the person as a whole: age, medical conditions, bad habits (smoking, drinking), type of work, and obesity. (However, there are studies in which it has not been proven that obesity is a contributory factor to have LBP.) Most textbooks mention a particular surgical technique for a determined spinal problem, but they do not refer to a specific patient with a unique condition or situation.

The physician should be aware of all circumstances when performing certain surgical procedures. There are occasions when the patient does not provide the physician with all the important factors and information necessary for the decision-making process. Patients should be thorough when answering questions while giving a medical history. In some instances, patients deliberately conceal certain information for several factors such as ignorance, secondary gain, and so forth. The surgeon should make a recommendation, but the patient should participate in the decision-making process. Making a decision for surgery on a patient with erroneous or incomplete information may create unfavorable consequences.

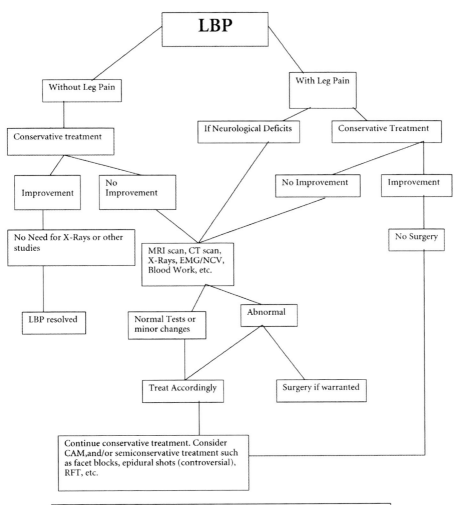

I created this simple flow chart. There are several Flow Charts that Institutions and Spine Centers have created; but one must tailor treatments to every patient.

Conservative Treatment. Conservative treatment for LBP typically involves bed rest, pain or muscle relaxant medications, and physical therapy. A back brace may be helpful. During physical therapy, ice or heat, acupuncture, chiropractic treatment, massage, TENS or PENS (transcutaneous or percutaneous electrical stimulation), ultrasound, and a program of low back exercises might be tried. There are studies in which TENS, ultrasound, and traction are not recommended for patients with LBP and muscle spasm. There can also be aquatic exercises (for example, hot tub and Jacuzzi) as part of the conservative treatment. Acupuncture is of no scientific value according to recent literature; however, some patients experience some improvement (possibly a placebo effect). Most recent publications mention massage as one of the only modalities of physical therapy with beneficial effect. A program of low back exercises (very specific) may be also extremely helpful, but one must be cautious because not all back exercises are beneficial for all patients with LBP.

I recommend restricting physical activity when there is an onset of LBP. I recommend avoiding bending, twisting, and lifting. Restrict sitting, walking, and standing for no more than twenty or thirty minutes a day. Patients should see me in two to three weeks or sooner if there are any symptoms of neurological deficits (for example, tingling, numbness, weakness, bladder or rectal dysfunction) after an onset of LBP. If there are neurological deficits, the patient should go to the nearest emergency department immediately.

Sometimes, I prescribe medications such as muscle relaxants, mild painkillers, and moist heat for twenty minutes two or three times per day for five to seven days. I do not recommend using ice; although, several studies recommend "first ice than heat." I have noticed different responses from patients; some feel better with ice but most feel better with heat. I tell my patients to use ice for the first twenty-four to forty-eight hours if they already used ice and felt better with it. If I see a patient within the first twenty-four or forty-eight hours after the onset of LBP, I recommend using heat. I do not recommend alternating ice and heat at any time. There can be muscle spasms and more pain if both temperature treatments are alternated. Applying warm cloths soaked in salty water to the lower back muscles may be comforting.

The myth of trying bed rest after an onset of LBP has been fading progressively and has been substituted by the most current agreement that patients should start early rehabilitation and be more active rather than sedentary. Trends in the treatment of certain ailments including the lower back have changed over time, sometimes contradicting the initial recommendation.

It is commonly agreed there is no need for bed rest even in the first stages of an acute onset of LBP. Once again, some of these studies do not separate LBP into categories. There are several causes of LBP. For instance, after an injury, a person with an onset of LBP may hurt more with movement if an extruded herniated disc is impinging the nerve root. Therefore, physical activity cannot only be painful, but it also increases the chances for nerve damage. The person with LBP should see a physician, preferably someone with experience, knowledge, and training in treating patients with lower back pain.

Some people like to have their spine adjusted or manipulated. These manipulations can actually be dangerous in some cases. The patient with fractures or neurological deficits should avoid strenuous therapy and activities that could cause further neurological damage and deficits. I would not recommend physical therapy for someone with a large herniated disc that is impinging on the spinal cord or nerves and causing neurological deficits such as weakness, numbness, severe radicular pain, or bladder or rectal dysfunction. I do not recommend physical therapy for a patient with a lateral or a far lateral herniated disc. These patients tend to have more than the usual pain for someone with a disc herniation. The disc fragment may migrate and intensify the pain and neurological deficits. Patients older than thirty or forty years of age should avoid spinal manipulations. It could be dangerous to wait for surgery and try conservative treatment first in some cases. Only the physician and, more specifically, a spine surgeon can establish if surgery or conservative treatment is in order.

A primary care physician, chiropractor, or other health care provider should have some basic knowledge in diagnosing and treating a patient with LBP. This diagnosis and treatment should be based on the history, exam, and radiological studies. A physician does not establish the best course of treatment without placing the patient at risk for complications if the physician bases treatment only on X-rays without a history and a physical exam.

A trial of conservative treatment is in order based mainly on the history and exam. The medical history plays an important role in the diagnosis and treatment of a patient with LBP. The physical exam is the complement of a medical history, and it plays an important role in the diagnosis and treatment of these patients as I mentioned previously. Radiological studies are taken into consideration during the diagnosis of a patient. A physician should decide if further tests are needed, and the patient should always be instructed that, if there is no improvement or if the condition gets progressively worse such as numbness, weakness, or bladder or rectal dysfunction, immediate medical care is mandatory. A consultation with a spine specialist may indicate emergency surgery is necessary.

Conservative treatment is recommended for patients that had an onset of mild LBP without neurological deficits or radicular pain. It is also recommended for patients who had certain studies such as a CT scan and/or MRI scan that indicated a mild bulging disc, moderate spinal stenosis, or osteoarthritis with some collapsing of the discs (not of the bones). Spine surgeons usually make the decision for surgical intervention. Therefore, the primary care physician will rely on the consultation with a spine surgeon. One of the most frequent mistakes physicians make is to believe that, with conservative treatment, surgery will always be avoided on patients with LBP. This information is erroneous.

Clinical studies have documented that as much as ninety percent of patients with LBP and a herniated disc in the lumbar spine improve without surgery. But, seventy to ninety percent of patients that have surgery have a favorable outcome (disc surgery).

Some studies lack certain comparative parameters. Furthermore, some studies have been carried out for only a short period. They do not follow these patients for several years. Many of the patients that initially improve with conservative treatment subsequently require surgery. They do not mention the percentage of patients that developed chronic LBP (or leg pain) because of late surgery. They do not mention the percentage of people that had complications during or after surgery (for example, dura tears, CSF leak, and nerve damage and chronic pain) due to adverse responses such as scar tissue formation after several months or years of trying "conservative treatment."

With these observations, I do not mean that all patients with a herniated disc should have surgery without a trial of conservative treatment. Actually, some patients not only improve clinically, but also resolve the disc herniation spontaneously. The disc heals and shrinks by itself without any particular treatment in some cases. Recent studies show shrinkage of disc herniation over time on MRI scan studies. I know patients who had a disc herniation in the lumbar spine by MRI scan and spontaneously improved (with or without "conservative treatment"). The MRI in some of these patients showed the disc herniation disappeared (that is, healed, shrank, or absorbed by itself). There is no clear evidence (studies) that a patient with an abnormal MRI scan of the lumbar spine will continue to get worse with time. However, common sense tells us a patient with risk factors for spinal deterioration (for example, heavy work, sports, smoking, and poor posture and body mechanics) will deteriorate further. One must be cautious when waiting for a herniated disc to "shrink or dissolve." Severe permanent neurological impairment may result from constant and prolonged nerve compression.

Clinically and practically speaking, there is not necessarily a need for more MRI scans if a patient with symptoms of LBP improves with conservative treatment. However, the real questions are: When will a herniated disc absorb spontaneously. If so, how long will it take for it to absorb? There is no clear data that demonstrates the percentage of spontaneous disc absorption and the factors that may influence this event (for example, locations of the disc, size, gender, and so forth).

Some studies have found that patients with sciatica also have concurrent bladder and rectal dysfunction (partial cauda equina) more often than physicians previously expected.

The number of people with sphincter dysfunction is underestimated. The same patient with a positive MRI scan indicating obvious pathology and the well-motivated person who had a reasonable trial of conservative treatment are good surgical candidates. The common recommendation for conservative treatment is four to six weeks.

How do physical activities such as physical therapy, tai chi, and meditation work? Do alternative medicine and physical therapy really help people with LBP get relief to the point of avoiding surgery? This is something that must be taken into careful consideration because there are applications for every treatment.

Physical therapy has mechanisms that help some people tolerate LBP:

- If the patient has a great deal of muscle spasm, using ice at the beginning followed by heat induces favorable relaxation of the muscle. Physical therapy is usually prescribed along with NSAIDs (nonsteroidal anti-inflammatory drugs). These drugs are usually used around the clock for the first three or four days instead of "on a PRN basis." One must be aware of the side effects and contraindications of NSAIDs, such as hypertension, history of peptic ulcer, bleeding disorders, and so forth.

- Exercises occupy the mind, distracting the pain receptors.

- Exercises increase endorphin levels, which are derivates of morphine. Under certain physiological circumstances, our body normally produces endorphins, which help deal with pain and other stressful situations.

- Exercise strengthens the muscles and stabilizes the spine. Endurance can also be increased as well as conditioning and fitness by exercising. I cannot overemphasize the multiple benefits of exercising.

Patients invariably ask me the same question: How can I exercise if I have pain in my lower back? Physical therapy has to be tailored for the patient's needs, size, age, and physical structure.

I have seen patients who received physical therapy for several weeks or months with no improvement. They also get addicted to pain medications when "conservative treatment" is extended more than eight weeks. When I asked what kind of physical therapy they had, they answer, "Well, I had some heat, ultrasound, and treadmill." Others said, "Treadmill, bicycle, massage, that's it." I think it is unfair to demand a patient lose weight before considering surgery. The reality is that the overweight patient will not lose weight soon and easily. These patients benefit from surgery when indicated. They should be treated as any other patient with LBP and a surgically treatable condition.

A problem exists with physical therapy in some settings. There seems to be no common agreement in the treatment of LBP, or perhaps the problem is that a physical therapist treats all patients with LBP the same way. I think this is a mistake, and it is the most frequent situation I encounter.

I have seen inefficient or partial physical therapy tried on patients receiving conservative treatment. Physical therapy was not tailored to the patient. There are also patients who are in "so much pain" that they cannot do anything and will not try physical therapy. Of course, one must first rule out a serious back problem. In my twenty years of experience, one of the most common mistakes I have observed is that physicians and patients take for granted a diagnosis and assume the "obvious."

The surgeon would say, "Well, the patient had a reasonable trial of conservative treatment and physical therapy, even epidural blocks. I think he or she is a surgical candidate." Nevertheless, the surgeon may have failed in getting a more detailed history and exam and in asking for the specific "conservative treatment" the patient was receiving. We assume the patient had the appropriate physical therapy and he or she failed it. Physicians do not wonder why the patient failed to improve with physical therapy and conservative treatment. Physical therapy may help or worsen the patient's condition. Conservative treatment (spinal manipulations, massage, ice, and so forth) may aggravate the back condition. Perhaps the patient did not have the appropriate therapy for the specific disorder. There is no specific rule for treating patients with LBP. One must first find out the cause of pain.

When using ice or heat during physical therapy, care should be taken to avoid direct contact with the skin. A wet towel or some kind of protection should be used to avoid direct contact because ice or heat can cause serious skin lesions (for example, frostbite, necrosis, and burns).

After twenty-four to forty-eight hours of "babying" the lower back, heat can be used following the same recommendations as for ice. Avoid direct contact, and remove the hot object immediately if you feel any discomfort. The heat may be used for only ten to fifteen minutes, but it can be used up to three or four times a day for another four to five days. Physical therapy can be started the first day with gentle massage and leg exercises.

I recommend physical therapy about two to three times per week for low back exercises, but the leg exercises, heat, and massage can be done every day. After a few days, ultrasound and TENS unit can also be added. Ultrasound can be used for no more than ten minutes, but the TENS unit can be used continuously as tolerated and based on the patient's response. Some people complain of more pain with the use of the ultrasound than with the TENS unit, heat, or ice. I recommend physical therapy for about four to eight weeks. I usually do not expect patients to notice significant improvement for the first two weeks of physical therapy.

Other types of physical therapy include (but are not limited to) pelvic traction, low back exercises, and manipulation. However, I do not recommend spinal adjustments or manipulations in some patients. I have redesigned some of the conventional low back exercises I believe are more beneficial and less stressful to the spine.

I have seen patients that respond very favorably to physical therapy even when they have moderate spinal stenosis. The downside is that, if they have spinal stenosis, chances are they will have only a moderate and temporary relief of the pain. Additionally, physical therapy is an alternative, and it is indicated for people who have medical problems that would contraindicate surgery or who may be at a high risk for surgical complications.

Walking is an excellent exercise, even if it is only a short walk. I do not recommend bending, lifting, or twisting the lower back. One must avoid all possible activities that could increase LBP. One must be cognizant of the need for a mattress that will suit a particular patient with LBP.

Along with physical therapy, other therapy techniques can be applied to patients—but again—only for certain spine conditions. Tai chi is an Oriental technique that has been used for several years not only to treat back pain, but also to treat hypertension, diabetes, rheumatism, weight control, emphysema, and other medical conditions.

What we currently call biofeedback is well known in Asian cultures. Some of these techniques are acupuncture, mental control, hypnosis, meditation, muscular exercises, and breathing exercises (yoga). Psychological therapy deals with stress and chronic pain. There is nothing wrong with massage and gentle adjustments, but one must be careful when a person is over thirty years of age because that person may already have degenerative disc disease (DDD). Brisk manipulations or adjustments may cause further damage on the already deteriorated disc.

The use of a low back support is also more of a myth. The industrial type, usually elastic, has been shown to provide no additional support to the spine. Its use is more psychological. It is a two-edged sword. The advantage could be that the back brace prevents a person from bending or stooping. The disadvantage may be that an individual feels confident the brace will protect him or her from injury and he or she may engage in more strenuous types of physical activities.

The use of a firm back brace (plastic or metallic) could be more efficient, but there is still controversy about it. Typically, the back brace is used for people who had a spinal fracture and do not necessarily require spinal surgery.

Some surgeons recommend the use of these braces for additional lower back support after surgery. Normally, it is after a spinal fusion intervention. The physician should be cautious when ordering a back brace because if the brace is used for more than four weeks, they can weaken the lower back muscles. This can cause even more pain to the patient. The recommended time for using the brace is also controversial. Some surgeons may recommend it for three, four, six, or eight weeks—and sometimes several months. There are patients whose spinal fusion does not "take," and the surgeon recommends using the brace for several months before another surgery is recommended.

Physical therapy is typically ordered three times per week for four to six or eight weeks. New data indicates some people may actually benefit with therapy two times a week instead of three times per week. Some surgeons recommend their patients with lower back conditions lose weight before even considering surgery.

Work hardening is a special program well known by physical therapists and physicians involved with patients that perform heavy work. This program is designed to encourage and help patients strengthen and condition muscles of the lower back for moderate to heavy work. The program is designed for certain patients. If care is not taken, patients not suitable for this kind of strenuous physical therapy may be hurt. The physician and patient must make the decision for a work hardening program. However, the physical therapist plays an important role in the development of the program. The patient should notify the therapist and physician immediately if there is any pain or discomfort with the program, so it can be discontinued at once. There is no obligation to continue or complete the program. Even for this program, I do not recommend bending and twisting the lower back. More importantly, I do not recommend lifting while bending or twisting the lower back.

One must be cautious with the use of NSAIDs and other drugs that may cause drug dependency. Certain side effects may also develop. The physician should be aware of drug interactions. The use of narcotic pain medication and muscle relaxants for more than three weeks should alert the physician that a more definitive treatment should be considered to avoid drug dependency. The physician should be cautious with the patient showing a drug-seeking personality or pattern. There is no medication that will replace physical therapy, meditation, and other nonpharmacologic treatments.

One has to remember that, in the process of becoming ill or healing, there is a fine line. Usually, the difference is in the balance of body physics and physiology. There is a significant "mind over matter" or psychological component in the process of developing an illness but also in the healing process. There are drugs that will mask pain and may even make matters worse.

Some psychologists and healers believe we bring disease and maladies upon ourselves because of inner psychological conflicts. It is a way of paying for situations we feel guilty about. Some people and physicians believe the body has the ability to heal spontaneously.

Although I recommend avoiding spinal manipulations on patients that have LBP associated with leg pain and/or neurological impairment, it has been published in the prestigious medical journals that chiropractic manipulations proved to be superior to conventional medicine when treating patient with LBP. One must be cautious, however, with spinal manipulation of patients older than forty years of age. A good chiropractor will advise the patient to avoid manipulations and get a medical evaluation if there is LBP that lingers for more than two weeks and if it is associated with leg pain, neurological impairment, weight loss, or some other ominous sign or symptom.

Semiconservative Treatment. These forms of treatment deserve to be further discussed. There are controversies related to the treatment of patients with LBP. Nonconservative, semiconservative, and alternative treatments involve:

- Epidural block
- Facet block
- Rhizotomy
- Selective nerve block
- Trigger point injection
- Adhenolysis
- Radiofrequency (RFTs)
- Implantation of pumps for pain control
- Nucleoplasty
- Percutaneous endoscopic discectomy
- Intradiscal electrothermal therapy (IDET)
- Spinal stimulator
- Chemonucleolysis
- Prolotherapy
- Others

These are procedures in which a physician—usually an anesthesiologist, neurosurgeon, orthopedic surgeon, or a physiatrist—treat patients with injections in different anatomical areas. A pain specialist not necessarily needs certification to practice pain management; however, physicians engaging in the practice of pain management are expected to be trained. They are also at least expected to take certification courses and seminars to be able to practice this medical discipline. It is expected, however, that pain specialists work with some limitations. For instance, it is not recommended a family practitioner, an occupational medicine physician, or a physiatrist performs invasive procedures such as spinal stimulator, pump implants, adhenolysis, and so forth. Some of these procedures could lead to serious complications. If they do, it is recommended they have the support of a spine surgeon in case of complications.

Epidural Injections or Blocks. Epidural injections or blocks involve the insertion of a spinal needle in the spine and over the dura, a sheet that covers the nerves and spinal cord (refer to anatomy). The difference is where the injection is administered. The injection can be applied in the center (middle) of the spine over the dura or on the side (transforaminal epidural block), close to the nerve that is pinched.

The needle may be directed to the joints, nerves, or ganglion of the nerves. Superficial injections may be given under the skin and in or over aching muscles. This procedure is called "trigger point injection." Usually, X-ray views are not necessary for the trigger point shots. However, X-ray visualization is required for other procedures (facet block, epidural block, rhizotomy, nerve block, and ganglion block). These are outpatient procedures unless the physician considers it necessary to stay for observation.

We must bear in mind the semialternative procedures involve potential complications. It is true that even conservative treatment such as physical therapy, massage, and exercises can aggravate the pain, cause nerve damage, and paralysis. However, when a practitioner starts introducing needles, probes, and other devices, devastating complications can occur. It is recommended the physician performing an invasive procedure in the spine have a spine surgeon available just in case there is a devastating complication (for example, hemorrhage, paralysis, infection, and so forth) in which emergency spine surgery could be required.

Complications can result from steroid medications with systemic reactions such as rash, allergic reaction, stomach or duodenal ulcer, osteoporosis, diabetes, and diabetic coma. They can also trigger diabetes on a person prone to develop it such on the obese person, the patient with history of diabetes, and the patient with Hispanic background. There may be reactions to the local anesthetic, allergic reactions, heart dysrhythmia, and so forth. The injection itself can cause nerve damage if applied too close to the nerves (chemical neuritis). There can be infection (superficial or deep) or bleeding (hematoma) that could lead to weakness or even paralysis. There can be pneumothorax (lung puncture) and other internal organ injuries (when injections are applied in the cervical or thoracic spine). There can be spillage of fluids or materials used for the procedures. These spills can occur around the spinal cord, and the complications can cause serious neurological deficits with complete paralysis (cauda equina syndrome) and bladder and rectal dysfunction. There can be severe pain and other unusual complications such as RSD (Reflex Sympathetic Dystrophy) or CRPS (Complex Regional Pain Syndrome). Other complications are tears of the dura and scar tissue formation, pseudomeningocele, CSF leak, headaches, meningitis, and needle breakage. Some rare cases have reported intracranial subdural hematoma and hydrocephalus. If the patient has an undiscovered brain tumor, applying a spinal needle can cause serious complications and even death. Fortunately, it is not common to have serious complications from epidural injections. It depends on the patient's reactions to the procedure and the physician's expertise

There are controversial results in studies about the use of epidural blocks ("cortisone shots") for LBP. Actually, there is a theory that steroids may hinder the normal healing process of the body by delaying the activity of macrophages, the cells responsible for immunity in the normal healing process. I have found that spinal injections can create scar tissue and cause further pain—not to mention the technical difficulty during surgery when surgeons struggle trying to release scar tissue from the nerves on patients who had conservative treatment for several weeks, months, or years. There are no studies that I am aware showing that epidural blocks cause epidural scar tissue formation; however, it is my observation there are patients in which scar tissue may develop after certain invasive procedures.

Patients with extruded discs may actually be more prone to have nerve damage by using cortisone shots that mask the pain. The patients may perform physical activities that could damage the nerve. There are physicians that will prescribe a trial conservative treatment with physical therapy and epidural blocks without radiological investigation for the cause of pain. On the other hand, there are patients whose symptoms and exam do not warrant expensive workup (MRI or CT scan), especially if the physician is relying on a "flowchart" or guideline.

If the studies are to be authorized by a health insurance, the representative authorizing tests and studies also relies on a guideline. Only if given certain information on the patient's condition, the insurance representative will make a medical decision. Sometimes, a person with no medical training will make decisions for treatment on patients with LBP. These decisions are related to the use of "cookbooks" or "guidelines" set in certain publications.

It is crucial a physician gets a thorough medical history and performs a meticulous exam. The physician should also be very familiar with some warning signs to look for during the examination of patients with LBP.

Epidural spinal injections can be considered on patients with severe LBP, osteoarthritis, or moderate spinal stenosis when surgery is contraindicated and when an epidural block is not contraindicated. However, I do not recommend epidural blocks for patients with severe spinal stenosis, osteoporosis, or medical conditions that could be complicated with the use of steroid medication.

We have to bear in mind that, if the spinal canal is already narrow and the nerves are squeezed or pinched, injecting a volume of fluid (local anesthetic, steroid drug, and saline solution) increases the pressure on the nerves and the chances for neurological deficits. Some may argue the volume of fluid injected is minimal, but it is still injected in a narrow space where there are nerves.

Epidural blocks on patients with moderate-sized bulging discs without herniation are controversial. These patients can be treated with noninvasive procedures such as physical therapy, medications, and other remedies. Some patients may benefit from the use of steroid. Steroids can also be used in a pill or patch form. It is not necessary to inject steroids in the spine.

I check the patient in a comprehensive manner and evaluate those with previous spine surgery and a history of peptic ulcer. I decide on an individual basis relying on the original spinal condition, medical history, exam, work history, social habits, and personality. Physical build (slim, medium, or obese) is also a factor in considering the different types of treatment. Other medical conditions, such as diabetes and use of blood thinners, may be contraindications for epidural blocks. Whoever does the procedure should explain the technique, indications, possible complications, expectations, and prognosis. When epidural injections are used, one typically applies the injections once every four to six weeks and only one to three times in six months because of the secondary effects. If the first epidural injection does not help, it is likely another one will not work either, but some clinicians give a trial of two to three injections (two or four weeks apart).

These are some of the invasive procedures used in semiconservative treatment:

IDET (Intradiscal Electrothermotherapy). IDET is a relatively new procedure in which a special wire or transducer is inserted in the disc through a needle. The procedure has been used for about a couple decades. The goal of the procedure is to "burn" the bulging part of the disc that is in contact with the nerve roots. Hopefully, with this procedure, the disc shrinks and heals, therefore releasing the pressure from the nerve. There are very satisfactory results from IDET, but only specifically selected patients are candidates for this procedure. Again, there can be complications from nerve damage, infection, and hemorrhage, including disc herniation if the disc was only bulging and not actually herniated. This procedure requires X-ray views. The patient may go home after the procedure, but the physician may sometimes want to keep the patient overnight for observation. As many other new procedures in the medical community, everyone wants to use it for most patients with LBP. Then researchers narrow down the use of procedures to only certain patients with certain clinical characteristics because of poor results on patients who did not need the procedure. Most recently, this procedure is losing advocates, and it has been decreasing in use.

Adhenolysis. Adhenolysis is a similar procedure requiring X-ray views during the process. A spinal needle is inserted in the area where scar tissue has formed. The goal is to "dissolve" scar tissue and separate it from the nerves. Some individuals tend to develop excessive scar tissue that can lead to chronic LBP. After inserting a spinal needle, a small catheter is introduced through the needle into the area of the scar, and saline solution is injected. There can also be complications such as infection, bleeding, and nerve damage with subsequent paralysis.

Spinal Stimulator. This is a procedure in which a special device, a spinal stimulator, is placed over the dura and out of the spinal cord. (Refer to the chapter in anatomy.) There are two or three incisions: one in the lower part of the upper back; the other incision(s) on the abdomen and side of the abdomen to place the spinal stimulator device under the skin on the abdomen area. The idea with this technique is to stimulate the spinal cord electrically, so the impulses will distract the pain receptors in the central nervous system and provide some relief. Typically, a trial device is attached to the patient's outer body. If the device results in pain relief, a permanent device is surgically inserted in the patient, and the actual stimulator is placed under the skin of the abdomen. Special care must be taken to avoid placing the device against a bony prominence. This can cause discomfort to the patient, not to mention other complications if the device is placed on other critical areas in the body. The procedure is done under X-ray view, and the patient may remain in the hospital overnight after the procedure for observation. This technique is usually recommended for patients who had extensive surgery, several operations, pain from spinal fusion hardware, scar tissue, chronic severe pain, and have not obtained pain relief with other conventional techniques such as physical therapy, exercises, and even epidural blocks.

If an MRI scan is ordered on a patient, the patient must notify the physician and the MRI technician that he or she has a metal device implanted inside his or her body such as a spinal stimulator or a pacemaker. It is contraindicated to perform an MRI scan on a person with metal inside the body. There can be serious complications.

Narcotic Pump Spinal Implants. Cancer patients may have severe spinal pain. A device called an implant or pump is positioned over the dura, outside the spinal cord. This pump is filled with narcotic pain medication so the patient can use it 24/7 directly in the spine area. The procedure is done under X-ray view. The patient may remain in the hospital overnight after the procedure. This procedure, as with spinal stimulator implants, can carry complications that can be devastating in some occasions such as infection, bleeding, neurological impairment (paralysis), meningitis, scar tissue formation, body rejection to foreign bodies, adverse reactions to medications, excessive drowsiness, respiratory depression, and even death.

Chemonucleolysis. This is a procedure that was used in the 1960s and 1970s with some degree of success. In this procedure, a special chemical is injected inside the disc. The principle was that the chemical would dissolve the herniated disc. Carica papaya, a proteolytic enzyme that "dissolves" the proteins of the disc, is the chemical used for the procedure. There were allergic reactions to it and even fatalities. The procedure lost advocates due to this complication. However, there have been new developments, and this procedure may gain more applications in the future. Physicians are starting to use this technique for patients with small protruding discs and no symptoms related to the protruding disc. This procedure is usually done under X-ray view on an outpatient basis.

Nucleoplasty. It is a relatively new, minimally invasive procedure in which radiofrequency (RF) is used to remove the nucleus pulposus material creating small channels within the disc.

Radiofrequency Treatments (RFTs). This is a technique in which the physician usually applies probes or electrodes close to the facet joints under X-ray view. Heat is applied over the joints with this device. The procedure ablates or destroys the small nerves attached to the joints. This technique is used mostly on patients with facet joint syndrome. This clinical diagnosis is often made by exclusion. Sometimes, prior to the RFT procedure, the physician injects the joints with local anesthetic and a steroid medication for diagnosis and treatment. If the patient gets some relief with the injection, chances are the patient will benefit with the RFT procedure. This procedure is usually done on an outpatient basis. The procedure may be repeated after a few weeks if the patient achieves some relief.

For a **Vertebroplasty,** cement is injected into the vertebral body. (Refer to anatomy of the vertebrae.) The problem with this technique is that the bone may collapse again. The procedure is similar to an IDET procedure previously described, but, in a vertebroplasty, the needle is applied in the vertebral body through the pedicle of the vertebra opposed to an IDET in which the needle is applied in the disc. This technique has been used also for vertebral fracture and collapsing of the vertebrae due to cancer and other conditions. The procedure can be performed on an outpatient basis, but the patient may stay overnight for observation and monitoring. Serious complications can occur, such as extravasation of the cement into the spinal canal and close to the spinal cord and nerves. There can be neurological impairment and embolism. There can be hemorrhage, infection, and other complications that can be devastating as in other invasive procedures.

Kyphoplasty is a newer technique than vertebroplasty. In kyphoplasty, the same principle is performed, but, in this case, a balloon is inserted in the vertebral body and then inflated. After that, cement-like material is injected into the vertebral body to maintain the shape of the bone and prevent the vertebra from collapsing again. These techniques are basically designed and intended to use on people with vertebral fractures (osteoporosis, cancer, and bone destruction). The complications are similar to the ones already described above.

What is a pain clinic? A pain clinic is a medical center or facility in which patients with pain (typically chronic pain) are treated. Anesthesiologists, physiatrists, orthopedic surgeons, and pain management specialists run these clinics. In these pain clinics, usually the patient with LBP is treated with invasive procedures such as epidural block, rhizotomy procedure, nerve block, IDET, spinal stimulator, spinal morphine pump implant, and so forth.

There is an American Board of Pain Management that certifies physicians (any specialty) to practice pain management. Physicians do not have to be certified by this board to practice pain management, but it is very helpful to take the courses to not only understand—but also to learn—the procedures typically used in the practice of pain management.

Epidural injections, trigger point injections, facet blocks, and other techniques used in pain management are only palliative measurements to control painful conditions, but there are spinal and medical conditions that simply have no cure. One must understand these injections may provide only temporary pain relief, but there is sometimes no improvement, and there can be complications with the applications of any of the pain management techniques.

There is the magic idea an injection will cure or help better than an oral medication. There is still in our culture the perception that injections have to be used to "cure" a condition. One must be cautious with this concept. One must also understand that epidural injections do not cure a medical condition. They may provide some pain relief sometimes, but it is my observation and experience that some of these procedures either do not help or have a placebo (refer to glossary) effect. Some patients experience even more pain. One, as a physician, must judge every case on an individual basis to use the best technique to help a particular patient. One must be honest when using some of these pain techniques. Physicians and patients frequently try to cure a condition the easy way: medications and injections.

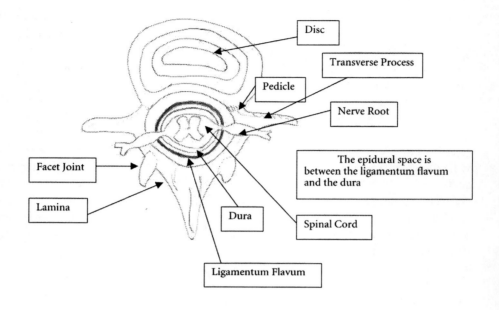

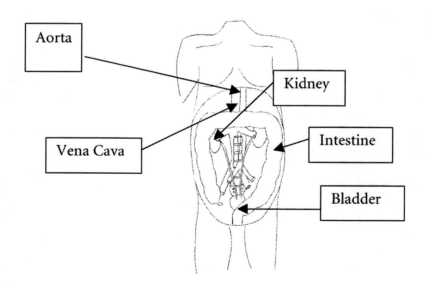

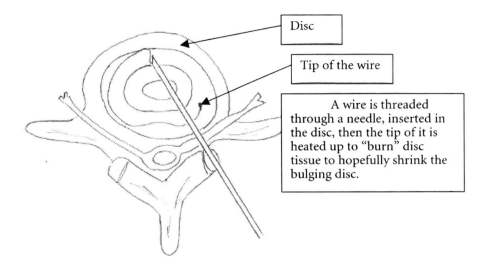

Disc

Tip of the wire

A wire is threaded through a needle, inserted in the disc, then the tip of it is heated up to "burn" disc tissue to hopefully shrink the bulging disc.

IDET (intradiscal electrothermal therapy) has been used as a semiconservative treatment for bulging disc that become symptomatic.

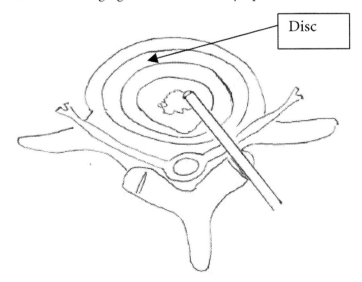

Disc

Nucleoplasty is a procedure in which the same technique for a discogram, endoscopic discectomy, and IDET is utilized. A needle or probe is inserted inside the disc under X-ray view. In the case of a nucleoplasty, the inside of the disc is "dissolved" with the use of radiofrequency (RF).

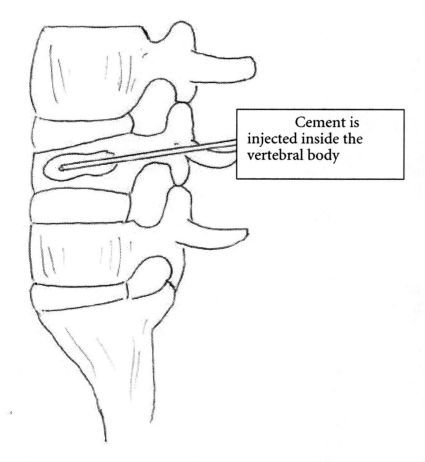

Cement is injected inside the vertebral body

A *kyphoplasty* is a procedure used for collapsing of the bones to restore the height of the bones by means of injecting cement inside the vertebral body. For a kyphoplasty, a balloon is applied inside the vertebral body to then inject cement. Whereas, in a vertebroplasty, only the cement is injected without expanding the vertebral body. These procedures are mostly used for patients with osteoporosis, but there are recent studies in which vertebroplasty was used for other causes of vertebral compression fracture. A needle is introduced into the vertebral body through the pedicle of the vertebra and under X-ray view.

Complementary and Alternative Medicine (CAM)

What is alternative medicine or holistic medicine? Alternative medicine was the first line of treatment for centuries until orthodox or modern medicine was introduced and more scientific medicine took over alternative medicine. To me, alternative medicine is the use of any kind of unorthodox or semi-orthodox (with partial scientific basis) remedy, cure, or healing technique applied to help improve or heal the body.

Alternative medicine has been regarded as a primitive, ignorant, old-fashioned practice of medicine. It is true fraudulent people and charlatans use these techniques to take advantage of desperately sick people. However, we have to remember there are also dishonest people in orthodox medicine who practice bad medicine. In general, dishonest people are in every profession. One of the reasons for distrusting alternative medicine is there is no clear scientific way of explaining the mechanism of action of these treatments.

However, it is well-known that some advances in medicine and other areas have been discovered by accident. While working on a medical project, an unexpected outcome resulted with significant implications. Modern medicine is full of incidental discoveries, for example, taking penicillin and the smallpox vaccine. Other discoveries were made while working on a project with entirely different results than expected.

More and more people are seeking remedies other than surgery for ailments including low back conditions. It has been estimated that, in the United States:

- 80 million people sought chiropractic treatment in one year for neck and back conditions
- 30 million people had massage therapy
- 20 million had energy therapy
- 20 million had relaxation techniques
- 10 million had yoga
- 20 million had other forms of complementary and alternative medicine (CAM)

It has been estimated that, between 1990 and 1997, from thirty-three to forty-two percent of Americans have turned to alternative medicine. In 1997, an average of eighty million Americans spent twenty-seven billion dollars in alternative medicine. One of the main reasons for turning to alternative medicine is the limitation of modern medicine to treat chronic or incurable ailments such as chronic pain, cancer, AIDS, and so forth. Against popular beliefs, Europe, particularly Germany, is one of the countries to use alternative medicine to an estimated sixty-five percent, followed by Sweden, France, Australia, and the United States.

Observation and human intuition have been the leading motivators when medical breakthroughs happened. It is not unusual to experiment with the result of an action first and then try to discover the cause or mechanism of the action. However, there is a logical and scientific explanation for how alternative medicine works. It is considered as such because no scientific data has been collected, but it does not mean it does not work. I have my own theories of how alternative medicine works, but I can expand on this subject in another publication.

Our body has its own healing systems that will help us recuperate and heal from a disease as animals when wounded or sick. Alternative medicine can work by boosting immunity to reach optimal health, changing bad habits, and making the body release certain chemicals to fight disease and painful conditions. The body is so wise that it can create its own analgesic substances to resist pain. Using our own body's powers and systems, alternative medicine works.

Alternative techniques have gained more popularity because of their benefit and have proven more effective than other conventional techniques. It requires a well-trained person to administer these treatments, and one should be aware of the charlatans and fraudulent practices.

Some health insurance companies will cover for certain management treatments, such as physical therapy, chiropractic manipulations, acupuncture, and so forth. However, many health insurance companies do not cover expenses for acupuncture treatments.

Many cultures and religious groups have used alternative medicine for centuries. Alternative medicine is not a new healing technique. These treatments are just surfacing in the western hemisphere, but, even in the old Indian cultures in America, rituals and healers used different techniques to heal people. Some of these techniques are connected with religious beliefs and rituals but based on simple principles.

- The patient must want to heal and do his or her part complying with the physician's recommendations (discipline) and must follow specific, ritual instructions and treatments.

- The healer should master alternative healing techniques.

- Any healing technique used on a patient should not cause more harm than the disease itself.

- I believe some disorders are related to the following factors: **Psychological.** There can be conscious or unconscious secondary gain because the patient is using the disease to attract sympathy and love (manipulative), and it is up to the individual to change attitudes and life perspectives and expectations. The mind is so powerful that it can attract diseases and heal. The subconscious mind works in ways to make the individual cause a disease. The mind may work as a way of punishment for feelings of guilt that may be related to childhood. These psychological traumas may form the future hypochondriac, chronically sick person, drug addict, alcoholic, and so forth. Daredevils may also fall into this group. **Ignorance** can be the cause of body harm. Our instincts alert us when danger is at hand, but we sometimes ignore these inner voices, instincts, or advice. Sometimes, true ignorance related to cause-effect situations or activities may be the reason for unfortunate events that lead to painful conditions that may last a lifetime. **Imbalance of the body fluids and energy and debilitating conditions.**

- **Destiny.** This is something very controversial, but there are mystical theories of reincarnation and a function in this life to suffer certain conditions to attain spirituality. Pain and suffering are used to purify the soul. There is a specific reason and goal for calamities that overwhelm us.
- **Genetic.** Some people have an adventurous personality. They will try high-risk enterprises.

In alternative medicine, as in orthodox medicine, some ingredients and rules should be followed and are vital to make medicine work:

- Faith
- Commitment
- Discipline
- Persistence
- Honesty
- Compliance

Alternative remedies may include (but are not limited to):

- Low back exercise
- Regular exercises (cardiovascular workout and endurance exercises)
- Physical therapy
- Chiropractic management
- Osteopathic treatments
- Cardiovascular activities (such as Stairmaster, bicycle, treadmill, walking, swimming, hiking, and so forth)

I personally recommend low back exercises, tai chi, and other Oriental disciplines. One must be cautious with strenuous martial arts and yoga.

These are some of the alternative medicine techniques used to heal the body:

- Hypnosis (and autohypnosis)

- Acupuncture, acupressure, Shiatsu, reflexology, massage
- Herbal remedies or herbal therapy, naturopathy
- Neural therapy
- Homeopathy
- Iridology
- Spiritual healing
- Chelating therapy
- Nutritional therapy, special diets
- Psychotherapy
- Biofeedback and psychological counseling
- Traditional Chinese Medicine
- Detoxification
- Environmental medicine
- Alphabiotics
- Reiki
- Flower essence
- Vitamin therapy
- Aromatherapy
- Meditation
- Polarity therapy
- Yoga, meditation, tai chi, Chung Moo Doe (not just any kind of martial arts or karate because some of these techniques could cause more damage if not done properly). I have read yoga is helpful for low back conditions. I would recommend being cautious specifically with yoga and certain martial arts because they can actually be more harmful and aggravate low back conditions. Remember that not all patients with LBP have the same illness.
- Ayurvedic medicine
- Radionics
- Breathing exercises
- Therapeutic touch
- Trager

- Animals and pets (dolphins, horses, dogs, birds, fish, and so forth)
- Color therapy
- Light therapy
- Use of magnetic devices
- Reading therapy
- Rebirthing
- Self-realization
- Invocations
- Past life therapy
- Affirmation
- Faith
- Dream work
- Healing angels/guides
- Spiritual blessings
- Religion (prayer)
- Creative visualization and activities
- Positive thinking exercises
- Helping others with worse conditions
- Vibration therapy, sound and music, mantras, praying, vocal sounds, Gregorian chants, New Age, music and other sounds (animals, nature, and so forth)
- Bodywork
- Craniosacral therapy
- Oxygen therapy
- Magnet and magnetic field therapy
- Flower essence
- Journalizing
- Folkloric medicine
- Energy Medicine
- Support groups
- Other techniques

There are special healing techniques, such as praying and cleansing of the spirit with herbs, water, metal, and fire. These practices are common in Mexico and Central and South American countries. They are called "curas, curaciones, or limpias" that can be translated as "cleansing against evil."

Some of these techniques are more accepted than others. There are several centers of alternative medicine. For more details on any of these treatments, the appropriate information can be obtained at any public library, the Internet, or bookstore. I do have certain preferences for alternative treatment for ailments related to LBP and other low back conditions. As there are different low back conditions, there are also different treatments. There are conditions in which certain treatments could actually aggravate the medical problem.

More scientific investigation is being carried out in the area of parapsychology, a relatively new field that combines medicine, psychology, psychiatry, and other investigative means to prove that certain "paranormal" activities exist. There is a more scientific approach to the unusual, unexpected, and paranormal phenomena. Attempts are made to scientifically prove some of these phenomena. Parapsychology is the link between orthodox medicine and alternative medicine and filters the superstition and popular belief without scientific bases. More serious scientific research is being carried out to try to determine which alternative medicine treatments could be valid. There is literature and books published with scientific evidence on the value of certain treatments with alternative medicine. Sometimes, better results were obtained with alternative medicine than with orthodox medicine. In fact, the use of both—orthodox and alternative medicine—has been found to boost the effect of certain modern medical treatments.

There is now scientific evidence of the healing power of prayer and animal contact (dolphins, horses, dogs). I recommend reading the appropriate literature related to these topics.

Some of my favorite recommendations of alternative medicine for a patient with LBP are:

- Hypnosis (and autohypnosis)
- Faith
- Prayer
- Physical therapy with very specific therapy tailored to the patient's needs, certain low back exercises, and specific exercises I have modified based on my own observations (found at the end of this book)
- Tai chi
- Massage

- Biofeedback
- Meditation
- Touch, massage, acupressure, reflexology, and Shiatsu
- Diet (weight control)
- Music and creative activities
- Herbal therapy
- Breathing exercises
- Animals and pets
- Positive thinking and exercising
- Helping others

For a definition or more explanation of the previously listed healing techniques, I suggest researching the proper sources of information.

I suggest using common sense when using techniques mentioned above for treatment of LBP. Keep in mind that most insurance companies do not cover most of these alternative treatments. Several insurance companies will cover osteopathic medicine, chiropractic therapy, massage, physical therapy, and acupuncture.

Be aware of reports on supplements and herbs that have been linked with serious complications including kidney and liver disease. Some supplements can cause heart disease and even death in some occasions. Consult with your primary care physician and make sure the physician or person using supplements and herbs is well aware of the effects of the remedies. Be aware of charlatans. Consult a knowledgeable physician specialized in complementary and alternative medicine (CAM).

Some of the supplements that have been found to have deleterious effects on people are:

- Kava
- Androstenedione
- Aristolochic Acid
- Chaparral
- Germander
- Comfrey
- Yohimbe
- Organ and glandular extracts
- Others

Herbs have been used for the treatment of LBP in general. Some of these herbs are:

- Horse chestnut
- Du huo
- Willow bark
- Cramp bark
- Black cohosh
- Frankincense

"Physical ailments can sooner or later affect the spirit or the soul. It is up to us to find strength within and to heal from the inside out."
M.A. Gutierrez, M.D.

Universal Code of Ethics of a Surgeon

These are some ethical rules and recommendations we pass onto other generations as we teach our specialty to young surgeons:

- Be honest and ethical with a patient when surgery is (or is not) indicated. Use basic medical knowledge and the current medical information as well as common sense and personal experience when recommending any treatment including surgery.

- Do not attempt a new procedure without appropriate training and/or supervision. Avoid difficult cases that we do not do on a regular basis, or at least notify the patient of this situation. There are conditions that are rare in nature and represent controversial conditions. Be honest about our capabilities and limitations. Explain the hospital's setting, capabilities, and limitations for elective cases. This does not necessarily apply to emergencies.

- Do surgical procedures in which we have training and experience. Be prepared to deal with intraoperative (hemorrhage, injury to other organs) and postoperative complications. At least be able to temporarily control the complication immediately until another physician or surgeon can assist to resolve the problem or complication. Surgeons say, "Do not even attempt to do a procedure unless you know how to solve the complication."

- Do not harm or cause more damage with surgery. We should try to avoid complications. As the saying goes among surgeons, "The only surgeon who does not have complications on his or her patients is the one who does not perform any surgery." There is always a chance for unexpected, unforeseen complications. There are also anatomical variants and patients that respond differently to surgery.

- Never assume anything in surgery. Count all instruments, gauzes, and other material used in surgery.

- Before surgery, always check X-rays, labs, medical records, side of the condition (right or left), and talk to the patient and family members before surgery for any last-minute questions.

- Do not shift responsibility to someone else (that is, another physician, nurses, or the anesthesiologist). Talk to other health care providers to avoid miscommunication or misunderstanding. Be sure who is doing what. Play it safe. Do not rush into surgery if there is a problem in any of the presurgical steps and checks.

- Avoid the "God Syndrome." We have limitations and cannot manage everything in medicine. Admit mistakes, but do not make them again. Be honest to the patient when it comes to complications. Get another opinion when there is a difficult case or when there is any doubt or controversy on the treatment selected.

- Follow the patient after surgery for a reasonable period, depending on the surgical procedure utilized. We consider postoperative period to be about three to six months after surgery. Take care of the patient's needs during the postoperative period. Generally, we refer the patient back to the primary physician for further nonsurgical supportive care. Typically, after a postoperative period, if no more surgical procedures are needed, a surgeon may discharge the patient. Assist the patient in getting further care if there has been a complication, poor outcome, or worsening symptoms. Be honest with the patient when explaining adverse results. Do not avoid responsibility by "brushing off" the patient.

- If possible during consultation and before surgery, explain to the patient and a family member or friend all aspects related to surgery. Use models, videos, or books so that the patient will clearly understand what is involved with the surgery. Explain expected postsurgical results, special care, rehabilitation, medications, their effect and adverse reactions, wound care, suture removal (if any), diet, exercise, physical activities, driving, traveling, sex, and so forth.

- Discuss financial arrangements for surgery only when the patient insists on talking about it. Notify the patient of all the possible separate charges related to the surgery. Recommend that patients speak with the representative in charge of financial arrangements, billing, insurance policies, and so forth.

- Document all information in writing.

Age is not necessarily a contraindication for surgery, but the chances for other medical conditions or complications increase with age. A frail, elderly individual may be more prone to infections (pneumonia, urinary and wound infection, and so forth), medication side effects, adverse reactions to anesthesia, and others. The patient must be part of the decision-making process.

History of Lumbar Disc Surgery

LBP and leg pain were well known to ancient physicians. However, it was not until 1774 that Dr. Cotugno found the sciatic nerve (pinched nerve) as a cause of LBP and leg pain. However, it was not until later that Dr. Virchow in Europe described a traumatic ruptured disc for the first time. In 1864, Lasègue described the clinical findings of the patient with sciatica. The first successful surgery for a ruptured disc was in 1908 by Dr. Oppenheim, a German physician. This surgery was done through a complete laminectomy. After him, other incidental ruptured discs were described in autopsies on people who died of other conditions. In 1929, Dr. Walter Dandy in the United States also made meaningful medical and surgical contributions not only in the surgery of disc herniation, but also in other areas of neurosurgery. Dr. Schmorl made contributions in spine surgery by describing disc pathology in a German publication in 1932. Drs. Mixter and Barr in 1934 published a paper in the *New England Journal of Medicine* in surgery for disc herniation. Surgery for the herniated disc via laminectomy changed little until 1972 when microsurgery and disc injection with chymopapain changed the approach to disc surgery, and, since then, other variants and new approaches have been developed. In 1975, the first percutaneous discectomy was performed.

Spinal fusion and instrumentation started as early as 1887 when Dr. Wilkins made the earliest report of a spinal internal fixation. In 1937, Dr. Venable introduced the use of a cobalt alloy called Vitallium that had been used for dental bracing and internal fixation of limb fractures. Stainless steel was also introduced in the 1930s and, later, titanium, which is currently used for pedicle screws. Subsequently, in 1948, Dr. King used pedicle screws for internal fixation of the spine. In 1963, Roy-Camille of Paris was the first one to connect the pedicle screws with plates and rods. Dr. Steffee started using pedicle screws in North America in 1984.

From 1972 to the present, there have been tremendous advances in the treatment of disc disorders. There has been a great deal of research on the intervertebral disc. There have been significant advances in the knowledge of the spine, particularly in the pathoanatomy, biomechanics (physics and biology), and genetics of the disc. However, we are still struggling to find the perfect treatment for the patient with LBP.

In this chapter, I would like to mention some of the most important issues related to surgery.

- Surgical indications, contraindications, timing, techniques
- The failed low back surgery
- Complications

One of the main indications for back surgery is LBP associated with leg pain (radiculopathy) or sciatica that persists for more than four to six weeks.

My personal impression and opinion is that, in general, more than ten percent of people with a lateral herniated disc larger than eight to ten millimeters will end up having surgery or other intervention or invasive procedure, mostly when a disc herniation is located at L4-5 (due to the narrow nature of this level).

I am not aware of a more specific study in which patients who had a lumbar herniated disc larger than eight to ten millimeters were followed for three to five years and did not require surgery. It was not until recently that studies have shown the true history of patients with a herniated disc, and some of these studies now mention the different outcomes related to the size and shape of the disc herniation. Patients with large herniated discs should require surgery soon if they are experiencing pain and neurological deficits.

In newer studies, there is a correlation of LBP, symptoms of nerve impingement (sciatica) with leg pain and other leg symptoms, and the size of the disc herniation related to indications and outcome of surgery. Most statistics have been inaccurate when speaking of patients with LBP and their treatment. This may alter the results of large population studies because all patients are placed under one LBP category.

There are different sizes and locations of disc herniation. I have had patients with a relatively small disc herniation, but I have also seen a fragment of disc in the foramen, the narrow orifice through which the nerve comes off the spinal canal. I have found a small fragment in a narrow location during surgery. These small pieces cause the patient a great deal of pain.

Therefore, it is unrealistic and unfair to classify all patients under one LBP category and recommend the same treatment to all. What about the patient with a "far lateral herniated disc" or with a free fragment? Patients with a far lateral disc herniation or free fragment (a piece of a ruptured disc that may be lodged in a small, enclosed anatomical area) may need surgery urgently because they are in excruciating pain and tend to have neurological deficits. These variants can cause symptoms and pain at a different intensity. Current studies mention that patients with a "free fragment" do not necessarily need emergency surgery.

There are different variants when evaluating a patient with a disc herniation in the lumbar spine, not to mention the characteristics and special circumstances of the patient. The size of the disc is important as well as the location, the possibility of anatomical variants such as a conjoined nerve root, the anatomical shape of the spinal canal (congenital stenosis), and the level of the disc herniation. It is not the same case when the disc herniation is located at L1-2 as at L4-5. The L4-5 spinal canal tends to be narrower at this level when compared to L1-2 or L5-S1, which are more "lenient" and accept a relatively large herniated disc because of the larger size of the spinal canal.

One, as a surgeon, must use caution when recommending surgery to a patient, especially when factors altering the response to the disease are involved. There are always going to be patients seeking secondary gain, litigious individuals, and those under workers' compensation. The physician treating the patient under workers' compensation must exercise caution. Physicians tend to distrust the patient under workers' compensation. It is not unusual these patients are mistreated because they are labeled as chronic complainers, fakers, and so forth. But, these patients often have a legitimate injury and require medical treatment and sometimes even timely surgery. These are some common steps, recommendations, and preparations before and after surgery. Some of these may vary because every institution and physician has his own preferences and policies.

Preparation for Low Back Surgery/Checking into the Hospital/The Day of Surgery

Usually, physicians order patients not to eat or drink anything after midnight if surgery has been scheduled for the morning (7:30 or 8:00 AM). The reason for doing surgery on an empty stomach is that, if a patient is placed under anesthesia, there can be vomiting or regurgitation and passage of liquids or food into the lungs during or after being under anesthesia. This situation can result in serious complications such as pneumonia and/or brain damage because of the lack of oxygen going into the brain (anoxia). I personally recommend that patients have a light diet the day before surgery to avoid bloating and constipation difficulties after surgery.

Sometimes, there can also be decreased bowel movement activity or even paralysis after surgery. This condition can lead to serious complications. Laxatives, plenty of fluids, and/or juices after surgery may avoid paralysis of the intestines that can lead to a series of adverse outcomes.

Narcotic pain medication, position for surgery, and anesthetics can cause paralysis of the intestine, and this can be manifested as bloating after surgery. The patient should notify nurses and physicians so that appropriate steps are taken to avoid complications from this condition.

The patient scheduled for surgery should quit smoking and drinking alcohol at least two weeks before surgery. I also recommend stop taking all blood thinners, anti-inflammatory medications, and aspirin (if possible) about two weeks before surgery after checking with your primary care physician.

Some patients require aspirin to prevent having a stroke or heart disease, but risks have to be considered by the primary care physicians, cardiologist (if any), and surgeon. Before surgery, patients must notify the surgeon of all medications and herbs they are taking.

It is always a good idea to bring the list or bottles of medications the patient takes regularly to the doctor's office or hospital. This must include aspirin, Tylenol, vitamins, herbs, prescription medications, and so forth.

The surgeon will inform the patient when to stop taking them and when to start them again. Some people need antibiotics before surgery, for instance, when the patient wears a prosthesis, a heart valve, or for other conditions (for example, immune-suppressed patients).

The risk of excessive bleeding as a complication increases during surgery if the patient fails to inform the surgeon of all medications he or she is taking. A patient with excessive hemorrhaging during surgery may require blood transfusions. That creates a risk of adverse or allergic reactions to the blood and infections such as AIDS and hepatitis. Other possible complications could be hypertension, stroke or myocardial infarction, renal failure, poor healing, and infection.

Sometimes, the surgeon anticipates a large amount of blood loss. Spinal instrumentation and fusion can be extensive, and patients may require a blood transfusion. The patient can arrange to save his or her own blood for transfusion if needed.

Some spine surgeons will not do surgery if patients are heavy smokers (more than one pack per day) or if they drink alcohol excessively. Occasionally, we order special tests on individuals with certain medical problems such as alcoholism (liver function), lung disease, or heavy smokers (spirometry, chest X-ray, blood gases, and other lung tests), kidney disease (renal function), etc.

Before surgery, I order routine blood work (CBC, blood chemistry), PTT, PT, bleeding time (when needed), urine, chest X-ray, and ECG. A cardiologic or pulmonary evaluation may be required before surgery, mostly on people with a cardiac history or older than fifty years of age.

Checking Into the Hospital. Hospitals require patients to register before surgery. During the registration, the patient's blood work, X-rays, and other labs are done. These tests can be done a few days before surgery so that they will more accurately reflect the patient's medical condition just before surgery.

Ask your physician any questions before surgery even if you think it is a "dumb" question. Do not hesitate to cancel the surgery if there are significant reasons, concerns, or any other issues. Try to get all family members and friends who will be seeing you after surgery to also speak with your doctor before surgery. It is always a good idea to have personal matters in order including a living will, power of attorney, and so forth.

I instruct out-of-town patients to bring their MRI scan films and any other study they had before surgery. I will not proceed with surgery until I have the films. I usually have the films with me because I leave them in my office after I discuss surgery with the patients.

Family members and friends are welcome to come to my office before or after surgery to discuss any questions they may have. I have found that people understand surgical procedures better when I use a spine model and textbooks for my explanation.

The Day of Surgery. Each hospital has its own policies, but all generally follows the same procedures. Patients usually arrive at the hospital between 6:00 or 7:00 AM morning, and surgery starts around 7:30 or 8:00 AM. If there is a specific medical condition, the physician might want to admit the patient the night before surgery for further preoperative testing.

Do not be surprised or upset if surgery is canceled just before the procedure. In some occasions, there are unforeseen situations such as emergencies, malfunctioning equipment, abnormal labs, recent infections the patient had, and so forth. Patients are prepared with an IV, and a nurse may ask additional questions and ask for a brief history of the medical condition, allergies to medications, antiseptics, surgical tape, and so forth.

The nurses, anesthesiologist, and physician check the surgical consent is signed. The patient may sign the consent for surgery at the surgeon's office. Hospitals have their own consent form for surgery and anesthesia or for any other procedure to be done. The physician's office staff and hospital verify the insurance information. Most insurance companies require notification or preauthorization for elective surgery; otherwise, they may not cover the expenses of the operation.

Some physicians may provide the patient with written instructions for surgery, or they may provide an educational booklet some medical associations prepare. These instructions may be related to hospital registration procedures or postoperative symptoms that could be expected. These instructions "walk" the patient through the process of surgery. Some physicians prescribe a sedative before surgery. It is natural to be nervous before surgery. Physicians, nurses, and other operating room personnel try to soothe the unfamiliar environment for the patient by conversing or simply explaining what to expect. I recommend taking a shower before surgery.

The position on the operating table for surgery varies. The anesthesiologist also "walks" the patient through the process of anesthesia. Ointment is placed after anesthesia and before surgery in the patient's eyes to cover them and avoid corneal abrasions during surgery. Sometimes, the eyes are also covered with gauze. The breathing tube (endotracheal tube or ETT) is secured to the area around the mouth with tape or other devices. After the patient is anesthetized, a Foley catheter is placed in the bladder. If the surgery will last more than two hours, some surgeons like to use the Foley catheter on their patients. This is not only to quantify intake and outtake of fluids, but a patient who is under anesthesia for more than two hours could make enough urine to cause pain and other physiological changes unpleasant for the patient when he or she wakes up from anesthesia. If a long procedure takes place, there can be damage to the bladder and kidneys due to excessive urine collection in the bladder. I usually discontinue the Foley catheter the day following surgery; some surgeons remove it right after surgery.

After surgery, patients are in pain. Sometimes, they have nausea and vomiting. Sometimes, getting up to urinate is very unpleasant. Sometimes, there is urinary retention right after surgery. Using a "straight catheter" while the patient is awake is also extremely unpleasant.

After the Foley catheter has been inserted in the bladder, the patient is turned over onto his or her belly (if having spine surgery to be done from the behind). The position for surgery may vary depending on the patient's size, type of surgery, and surgeon's preference.

The surgeon must have explained—either in the office or just before surgery—the procedure he or she will be doing, indications, success rate, plus the most frequent and chances for complications so that the patient can sign a surgical consent. If there are some possible variants of the surgery (such as the use of hardware, plates, screws, surgery at other levels, fusion operations, and so forth), the surgeon should explained in detail these variations of surgery.

There is usually another consent for anesthesia the patient needs to sign. After the patient has been placed under anesthesia, the knees are bent, and the areas of the body that may be under pressure, such as bony prominence, should be padded to avoid sores or pressure on the nerves that could cause postoperative paralysis. The eyes should be free because pressure in the eyes could cause eye damage and blindness. The genitals should be free (male) and under no pressure. The surgery may take anywhere from forty-five minutes to several hours (six or eight), depending on the surgical technique to be carried out.

Prophylactic antibiotics (antibiotics given to prevent infection) are used sometimes before, during, or after surgery. Other medications may be used during surgery, depending on the medications the patient was taking before surgery.

The anesthesiologist monitors vital signs, oxygen saturation in blood, and other parameters. The anesthesiologist notifies the surgeon if problems arise with any of the parameters, for example, blood pressure, breathing tube, and so forth. The surgeon notifies the anesthesiologist of the surgical progress, bleeding during surgery, and how much more time is needed to complete the surgery. Blood loss is carefully quantified during surgery. Gauzes and instruments used in surgery are carefully counted before and after surgery. These observations are routine and very critical.

It is important the physician (surgeon) be informed before surgery if there is a prostate problem. The surgeon will be prepared to call the urologist to insert a Foley catheter on the patient before surgery.

After Surgery. The patient is awakened by the anesthesiologist (all anesthetics are reversed) right after surgery, and the breathing tube is removed (if possible). Suction is applied to the mouth to prevent any saliva from going into the lungs.

The patient is turned on the side if vomiting. (There is a taste in the mouth and a smell from the anesthesia that may be nauseating.) The eye ointment will be wiped off. There may be a piece of gauze or a sponge placed in the mouth before or during surgery to avoid biting the tongue, sticky pads on the chest from the intraoperative EKG monitoring, and a black, sticky strip on the forehead from the intraoperative thermometer.

Most of the time, the patient is disoriented from the effects of the anesthesia. But, in the recovery room, the physicians and nurses may be asking the patient to respond to some simple questions and commands: Are you in pain? Wiggle your toes for me. Move your legs or arms. There is a sensation of urinary urgency if a Foley catheter has been used. Patients are sometimes restrained if they become agitated from the anesthesia because they may start pulling the IV and urinary catheter. Pulling the Foley catheter while the holding or locking balloon is still inflated inside the bladder can cause other complications such as urethra lacerations.

The patient remains in the recovery room until he or she is stable (vital signs, neurological and cardiac status). Then the patient is sent to the regular floor or ICU if certain medical complications may be expected or if the patient had to remain intubated. Some patients react to anesthesia with disorientation, confusion, and even hallucinations. The elderly tend to have more effects related to anesthesia than younger patients; therefore, these patients may have to be restrained and placed on certain medications until the anesthetic wears off. This anesthesia-related confusion might last a couple of days or more.

After surgery, the physician typically writes postoperative orders. He or she may dictate the procedure to sign it later. Next the surgeon or assistant usually talks to the family about how the surgery went and expected postoperative outcome. The patient may remain in the hospital from one to two days or sometimes more, depending on the type of surgery and if complications developed.

If there was a spinal fluid leak as a complication during surgery, the patient may be asked to stay additional time in the hospital and remain flat in bed. Sometimes, a spinal catheter is applied to drain some spinal fluid and allow the leak to seal and heal. The surgeon will explain the seriousness of the complication, what to expect, and how to treat it.

The patient is entitled to ask all questions he or she may have related to the surgery. The surgeon will explain the findings of the surgery once the patient is fully awake from anesthesia. This may take a couple of hours or more.

The patient is placed on pain medication, such as a "PCA pump" or IV drugs. A PCA pump is a machine that precisely pumps pain medication into the patient's veins via a small button hooked to a machine.

The machine (pump) is set by the nurse to administer only the dose of medication ordered by the physician. The patient cannot be overmedicated because the pump has been preset. Only a specified amount of medication can be provided over a particular period.

Doses of medication for the elderly have to be adjusted because an elderly patient typically requires less medication for pain control. Regular doses of pain medication on the elderly could be dangerous, making patients excessively drowsy, which could also lead to respiratory failure.

Sometimes, the surgeon prefers to use pain medication around the clock, for instance: Morphine 2 mg IV, SC or IM every two to four hours or Demerol 25 or 50 mg IV or IM every three to four hours. Different pain medications are used after surgery. The surgeon will encourage the patient to take oral medication as soon as an oral diet is tolerated. I recommend taking the oral form if IV medications have been used after surgery. IV medication may cause local irritation of the veins and other reactions. The IV medications also tend to be more expensive than the oral form.

The diet is started after surgery only if the patient is fully awake and oriented, if there is no nausea or vomiting, and if there is bowel activity (checked with a stethoscope by a nurse or doctor). The diet can be liquid, soft, or regular, depending on the patient's tolerance, bowel activity, and the surgeon's orders.

The Foley catheter is usually removed the same day of the surgery or the following day. A foreign body (catheter) can cause a urinary infection if it is left in the bladder several hours or days.

The trauma of surgery can be the reason for low-grade temperature after surgery, as well as anesthesia, room temperature, blood absorption, or other factors. The anesthesiologist and/or the surgeon encourage the patient to use an incentive spirometry, which is a device used for suction to keep the lungs expanded because atelectasis (collapsing of the lungs) is one of the most frequent causes of postoperative fever. Atelectasis may progress to pneumonia if not prevented or treated. However, one must be aware of CSF leak and not use incentive spirometry enthusiastically after surgery because this therapy worsens CSF leaks by increasing the pressure inside the veins and spine.

The dressing is usually changed the same day, day after surgery, or as needed if there is too much drainage. A nurse usually changes the dressing. The surgeon may want to inspect the incision the day following surgery.

Usually, I order physical therapy after surgery, mostly to have the therapist teach simple, easy low back exercises the patient can do in bed and later at home. The therapist will also educate the patient in activities, getting off and on the bed, as well as activities of daily living (ADLs). The patient is asked to get up and try to walk the next day after surgery if there have not been any complications. The therapist instructs the patient in body mechanics and passive exercises for the extremities.

How long will I stay in the hospital after back surgery? My patients ask this common question. The length of hospital stay varies. Each surgeon has his or her own preference. It also depends on the kind of surgery performed, the age of the patient, medical condition, complications, and so forth. I usually keep patients in the hospital from one to three days. It is rare I keep them longer than three days. Some patients feel we, surgeons, sometimes want to send them home "too soon" because we want to please the insurance companies to save financial resources. I explain to patients that it is not "too soon." It is simply indicated to send them home. The less time they spend in the hospital, the less chance they have to catch infections from other patients. Hospitals can also be noisy. Or simply, nurses awaken patients every certain time to take vital signs and for checking on other patients. I strongly believe patients recover better at home in their own environment. In some occasions, such as when I have elderly patients, I send them to an in-house rehabilitation center. Home health care can also be used to assist patients at home.

The patient may be discharged if he or she is:

- Eating well
- Urinating
- Having a bowel movement or bowel activity
- Walking independently or with the use of assistive devices
- Taking oral medications
- Having good pain control with oral medications
- Improved from the symptoms (One must bear in mind there is sometimes no immediate improvement of symptoms after surgery for a number of reasons. The surgeon will explain them and will decide if the patient is ready to go home.)

Also, the patient can be discharged:

- If the incision is in good condition
- If the vital signs are stable and there is no fever
- If certain previous medical conditions particular to the patient may have been stabilized
- If arrangements for ADLs or transfer to a rehabilitation center have been made
- If the patient has understood postoperative care and instructions for physical activities
- If there is a person responsible for transporting the patient after surgery

The patient is then discharged with prescriptions, physical therapy booklets, and other instructions from the physician. There are surgeons who perform back surgery on an outpatient basis.

The surgeon usually gives the patient an appointment for a postoperative follow- up that may be in two or three weeks or later. The patient should notify the physician at any time before the appointment if there has been a problem with the surgery. If there is an alarming sign or symptom, the patient should go to the emergency room so that the surgeon (or the covering physician) will be called in. Some patients will need a back brace after surgery. The surgeon will make recommendations depending on the type of surgery.

It is a good idea to make arrangements for personal items and other personal affairs before surgery (living trust, a will, life support instructions, etc). No matter how meticulous a physician is and how extensive the cardiac and medical workup was made to optimize the patient for surgery, patients can have postoperative complications that can sometimes be devastating (stroke, heart attack, pneumonia, etc). Complications can cause brain damage and even death.

Arrangements for a ride after surgery should have been made. There is a good chance the patient may have to lie down instead of sitting up during the ride back home. Some people use a van, minivan, SUV, or vehicle in which the front seat can recline all the way down or in which the backseat can be used to lie down. It is better to avoid bumpy rides. Generally, the patient will not be able to drive for about two or three weeks, depending on the procedure performed.

It helps to arrange for home equipment, hospital bed, braces, a raised toilet seat, stools, cane, walker, and so forth before surgery. It is better to stay on a ground floor for the first two or three weeks after surgery. Before surgery, be sure to get plenty of food supplies and other items such as a flashlight, matches, candles, and telephone nearby to be prepared when the patient returns home after the operation.

It is a good idea to wear slip-on shoes and clothing that is easy to put on and take off. I advise patients to quit smoking after surgery. Smoking can increase the chances for respiratory complications, such as atelectasis, bronchitis, pneumonia, and infection. I also advise patients to take plenty of fluids and laxatives if necessary after surgery.

Constipation is expected because of inactivity, pain medications, and the use of anesthesia. Most narcotic medications will cause constipation. Use a stool softener for constipation to decrease straining.

Ask your surgeon about sex. Usually, common sense will give the patient a hint on physical activities the body will tolerate. If the patient is in a lot of pain, any strenuous physical activity should be avoided. About two or three weeks after surgery, the patient may want to have sex. Ask your surgeon about it. Try to use a comfortable position. Do not engage in any awkward positions. Do not bend or lift. Lie down on your back, and do not remain in an uncomfortable position. Let your partner do most of the work at the beginning. Use a position that will keep your back safe during sex.

Sometimes, the surgeon uses stitches or staples to close the wound. The sutures will have to be removed in about two or three weeks, depending on the surgeon's instructions. Usually, the surgeon will have a nurse or someone in his or her office remove the sutures or staples after surgery. I strongly recommend the surgeon give the patient a card indicating the surgical procedure, making it available when he or she sees another physician. I recommend avoiding straining, bending, lifting, twisting, driving, climbing stairs, and riding in vehicles for at least the first three weeks. Avoid bending and twisting permanently.

Make sure you understand body mechanics after surgery, physical therapy, exercises, and instructions for taking a shower. Change the dressing every day.

Have someone inspect the wound. It is normal to have a little discharge through the wound at first. This may be related to the irrigation of sterile water used during surgery. Itching around the incision is normal. This can be from the antiseptics used or the healing process. The incision may start to look white and will start making a scab. This is all normal. What is not normal is redness, swelling, and increased temperature around the wound. Fever can also be a sign of infection. Increased back pain can be due to a smoldering infection that can be superficial, deep, or both. Increased back pain, leg pain, and fever may be a deep infection in the disc space. The surgeon must be notified of any of these signs and symptoms as soon as possible.

I have noticed two extremes in patients: the patients who do not want to bother the physician with "dumb" questions and the ones that ask every simple question. Some patients do not read the written postoperative instructions, they lose them, they do not understand them, or they simply wanted to "touch bases." These two extremes may lead to misunderstandings. Serious problems may develop (infection, hemorrhage, heart attack, and so forth) after surgery. The physician must be aware of these situations.

Sometimes, physicians have a physician assistant or nurse practitioner that will answer the calls, but the surgeon may respond first if he or she considers the patient could be at a high risk for complications after surgery.

If you call your surgeon and receive no response from him or her or the office on the same day, call the physician again. Do not wait until the next day to get an answer. Inform the answering person or system that it is important you speak with your surgeon.

If you still did not get through to your surgeon, go to the local emergency room. If the on-duty physician considers your complaint or problem critical, he or she will call your surgeon. If your surgeon is not on duty, the emergency room physician should call the on-duty one covering for your physician. This physician should be able to evaluate and determine the reason for your concerns.

If for any reason there is no way to reach your surgeon or primary care physician, the emergency room physician should resolve the problem by sending you to another facility or another surgeon if necessary. (This is the extreme.) Usually, the issue will be resolved without these extreme measures.

It can be alarming and may create anxiety for the patient if, after surgery, there is a new symptom(s) not present before surgery (numbness, weakness, or pain). Your surgeon must explain the possible causes of these situations.

After surgery, you are expected to do some light leg exercises maintaining the lower back. Always lay flat, avoiding twisting and bending it. Avoid climbing ladders or stairs, walking on inclinations, or driving. Read your physician's instructions if given to you.

I recommend physical therapy three weeks after the surgery. This first three weeks are for recovery and healing. Usually, patients cannot drive or ride for this first three weeks. I recommend physical therapy three times per week for four, six, or eight weeks, depending on the patient's response and motivation to physical therapy. I usually explain what to expect from physical therapy and what not to do or expect from it. It is my preference to give specific instructions to the therapist for the physical therapy. It is never expected to have more pain with physical therapy. "No pain, no gain" does not apply to patients with LBP. Avoid bending and twisting the waist as well as lifting more than five pounds.

It is better to avoid sitting for more than fifteen minutes at a time after surgery. Sometimes, people tend to develop muscle spasms that become severe. Sometimes, there is pain radiating down the leg, just as before surgery. This can be due to muscle spasm and nerve swelling. The patient panics because of the severe pain developed after surgery and it takes a good while to get over the muscle spasm. However, in some cases, a fragment of disc could have migrated after surgery, or there may be a brewing infection or a hematoma (blood clot) that could cause recurrent leg pain. One must be cautious with certain symptoms that develop after surgery.

Postoperative Care After Your Low Back Surgery and Other Recommendations Before and After Surgery

These are written instructions I give to my patients before surgery:

Activity. For the first two weeks, I recommend restricting standing, walking, and sitting for only up to twenty minutes at one time. However, easy, simple physical activities are encouraged to prevent urinary infections, pneumonia, and blood clot formation in the leg veins. It is better to walk for a few minutes two or three times a day than to walk more than twenty minutes at a time during the day. Light physical activity, such as walking, benefits the healing process by increasing blood flow to the wound and decreasing the chances for infection. Walking and easy low back exercises also decrease muscle spasm and pain that may develop after surgery.

Using common sense, progressively increase exercises and physical activity. Do not stand or sit in one position for more than fifteen minutes at a time for the first three or four weeks after surgery. Frequently, while in the hospital, a physical therapist sees the patient for instructions on physical activities such as getting in and out of bed, log roll, balance, and so forth.

Sometimes, the therapist teaches the patient simple leg, hip, knee, and low back exercises that I encourage they continue doing at home. The surgeon may have a sheet, pamphlet, or brochure with some exercises to do at home. I recommend keeping the head of the bed either flat or elevated up to only thirty degrees when sleeping. The average head elevation is about twenty degrees.

It is better to use a pillow for support between the legs at first. Sometimes, it is more comfortable to place a pillow under the knees. When getting up from lying down, log roll on the side, swing the legs around, and then come up with the upper body as one unit while letting the legs come down to the floor. Use the elbows and arms. Use the heels for leverage to move in bed when laying flat on the back.

Occasionally, a walker or a cane may be necessary. Ask the therapist and physician about it. Do not drive or ride vehicles for at least the first three weeks. Avoid slippery or wet floors and stairs or any surface where the patient may trip and fall.

Adapt the house and bed for after surgery (for example, get objects close to the bed, bring objects down from heights, wear loose-fitting clothes that are easy to put on and take off, use sandals or slip-on shoes, and so forth). Do not climb ladders, and, if it is necessary to walk up or down the stairs, do it slowly and carefully to avoid a fall.

Wound Care. Most of the time, I suture the wound from the inside with absorbable sutures. They will absorb, and the knot will fall out in about three weeks. Some surgeons use sutures (stitches) and some others use staples. Sutures or staples need to be removed about two or three weeks after surgery. It is normal to itch in the area of the surgical wound; this could be related to the antiseptic used to clean the skin before surgery and to the healing process. Sometimes, a skin reaction with redness and even blister formation occurs with the use of certain surgical tape. It is better to use paper surgical tape than the silk type.

Do not apply any ointment or lotion on the wound for the first two to three weeks. Change the dressing every day without touching the wound. I recommend using a clean plastic bag cut in half and taped across the upper back to cover the wound when taking a shower. Use assistance, and sit in a plastic chair when taking a shower. If the gauze accidentally gets wet, simply replace it with new and clean gauze. Check the wound every day, and change the dressing. It is normal to see a fine, white line in the middle of the wound. It means it is already healing. Leakage of "watermelon-like" drainage for the first two or three days is normal. Simply change the dressing. This is usually residual water used for irrigation during surgery that possibly stayed deep inside the wound, and, when applying pressure on it (as when lying down), the fluid seeps out.

There may be some swelling and redness around the wound and muscle spasms (pain and swelling) during the first two or three weeks. Leave the wound and surrounding area alone, or use a heating pad for up to ten minutes on the sides of the wound (but not over the wound) two or three times per day for two or three weeks. Do not apply the pad close to the wound or burn the skin with it. Do not sleep on a heating pad.

I prefer that ice be avoided. Do not scratch on or around the wound. Usually, when the wound has been closed from the inside, there are "steri-strips" that hold the skin together. Do not remove them for the first three weeks. At the end of the three weeks, take a regular shower, get the wound wet, and peel off the "steri-strips" carefully. Dressings will not be needed after that. It is okay if the "steri-strips" come off before three weeks. Just keep the wound clean. If there are sutures on the outside of the skin, the sutures have to be removed in about two weeks after surgery.

Signs of infection would be increased drainage, bad odor, yellow or green drainage, redness, swelling, and severe pain. There can also be fever, chills, night sweats, headaches, nausea and vomiting, neck stiffness, and generalized weakness. Contact the physician (surgeon, the primary care physician, or the emergency room). Infections can occur at different levels:

- Skin infection or wound infection (superficial infection)
- Deep wound infection or infection of the fascia, muscles, and soft tissues
- Deeper infection involving the bones and/or discs
- Systemic infection
- Meningitis (if there has been a CSF leak)

Temperature. The trauma of the surgery usually develops a low-grade temperature around 99 and 100.5 degrees for the first few days. The body metabolism also increases. What is not expected is a temperature over 100.5 for more than two or three days. This low-grade fever can be related to a number of causes. It does not necessarily mean there is a wound infection. In fact, most of the time, lung congestion causes fever after surgery.

Use of Incentive Spirometry. The use of incentive spirometry is very important after surgery. It can prevent pneumonia and other lung-related complications. The "I.S." is a plastic container with a short, blue hose or pipe in which the patient suctions as much as possible to maintain the lungs inflated. I recommend using it two or three times every two to three hours after surgery when the patient is awake (daytime). After surgery, patients tend to develop atelectasis, which is the congestion and collapsing of the lungs. This condition can progress to pneumonia if the I.S. is not used. Smokers are more prone to develop these complications. However, if there is a temperature of more than 101 degrees, notify the surgeon or the primary care physician or go to the emergency room.

Diet. The patient is not to eat or drink anything after midnight the day before surgery. Fluids or food may be aspirated into the lungs during anesthesia if he or she drinks or eats a few hours before surgery. I recommend a soft diet after surgery for the first three to five days to avoid constipation and abdominal pain or discomfort

The use of anesthetics and pain medications cause the intestine to function more slowly. Sometimes, the intestine paralyzes, and serious complications such as bowel distension and rupture can occur. If bloating, abdominal pain, nausea, and vomiting increase, the patient must notify the surgeon or primary care physician or go to the emergency room.

I recommend eating a light and soft diet before surgery. Frequently, it is necessary to use mild laxatives such as milk of magnesia, Dulcolax, Colace, Metamucil, and other laxatives because constipation is very common before and after surgery. Drink plenty of fluids including prune juice, orange juice, or any other drink. Eat fruit, cereal, bran, or food the patient is familiar with and has used before for constipation. If you are diabetic, keep your diet as indicated by your primary physician.

Avoid using long-term narcotic pain medication, and try to substitute or alternate with other nonnarcotic medications such as ibuprofen or Tylenol. If the patient was on a special diet before surgery (for instance, diabetics and kidney failure patients), resume that diet. Try to take pain medications with meals to avoid stomach irritation. Sometimes, the physician will prescribe an antacid to avoid gastritis or peptic ulcer.

Medication. Continue taking medications taken before surgery for medical conditions as prescribed by the primary care physician (such as blood pressure medications, heart medication, insulin, Synthroid, and so forth), unless instructed otherwise.

Use only the anti-inflammatory and pain medications recommended and prescribed by the surgeon upon discharge. Stop taking any other pain medication or anti-inflammatory medications taken before surgery. Try not to take more than one anti-inflammatory medication because they can cause serious upper gastric hemorrhage, gastritis, or ulcer.

I have had excellent results using antibiotics to avoid infection, although their use is controversial for "prophylactic" reasons. Sometimes, when a bladder infection is suspected, I prescribe the antibiotic Keflex, Levaquin, or Cipro before surgery. The patient should continue to take it after being discharged from the hospital. I definitely use antibiotics on diabetics and debilitated patients who may be prone to infections. One must be cautious on patients prone to bleeding because some of the above antibiotics can cause a postoperative hemorrhage.

It is generally recommended not using antibiotics for surgery because there is theoretically no need for them if the surgery was performed under sterile technique. However, some surgeons prefer to use antibiotics before, during, and after surgery. Especially if the surgery was long, there was the possibility of contamination of the wound by the use of the microscope, new operating room personnel, or on a patient that may be prone to infections.

I usually prescribe pain medications for surgical patients. Most of the pain medications on the market are narcotics and can have minor, mild, or serious side effects. The most common reactions I have seen in patients are constipation, itching, restlessness, and nightmares. Most of the pain medications are similar but come in different strengths. Morphine and Demerol are not necessarily the strongest pain medications. Each patient responds differently to medications. Those resistant to morphine or Demerol may get more pain relief with ibuprofen.

Sometimes, I prescribe one medication, but I may change it if there is an adverse reaction or they do not "take the edge off." Upon discharge from the hospital, I usually prescribe enough medication to last for about two weeks (thirty to forty pills). I do not prescribe large quantities of narcotic pain medication.

I suggest that, if a patient is running out of medication, the patient must call the office before 12:00 PM by Friday for a refill or for a new prescription. Some pain medications can be refilled over the phone, but others require a written prescription. New laws require physicians see the patient in the office if prescribing narcotic pain medication in some states.

Pain medications are addictive, as most people know. There can be other side effects, such as drowsiness, itching, nightmares, palpitations, dizziness, upset stomach, constipation, and so forth. Stop taking them if there are any side effects, and contact the physician(s).

Avoid excessive pain medication, and do not drink alcohol or take other sleeping pills at the same time. These combinations could cause serious respiratory depression, unconsciousness, and even death. Do not mix narcotic pain medications with sedatives or antihistamines (allergy medication) or medications that could cause drowsiness. Try to taper yourself off pain medications over time, as you feel less pain.

The patient must stop taking aspirin and anti-inflammatory medications before and after surgery because they increase the chances for bleeding during and after surgery. If aspirin is taking for a heart condition, notify the surgeon for specific recommendations for its use.

Bring a list of medications or the medication the patient is taking to the hospital so that the physicians and nurses will control the use of medications. It may be less expensive to use your own medications than those provided by the hospital.

Follow-up Appointment. When the patient picks up the preadmission papers from the office, the receptionist also has the postsurgery follow-up appointment date scheduled. Usually, the appointment is scheduled for about three weeks after surgery. It usually takes patients three weeks to recover from surgery. They can travel by car without much discomfort. Depending on certain circumstances, the surgeon may change the appointment date to before or after three weeks.

Possible Symptoms Experienced After Surgery. There are times when the patient feels immediate relief of the leg pain (if there was any leg pain before surgery) as well as times when no relief is gained. It is less frequent to have increased leg pain after surgery. Although, it is possible if there was some nerve manipulation removing a disc fragment or other unavoidable manipulation during surgery. There are times when there is also resolution or a new onset of numbness. This is rather alarming for the patient, but it is generally related to the same reason given above. Most of the time, these symptoms will resolve.

There is no specific time for the resolution of symptoms. It can be days, weeks, or months. Sometimes, the leg pain goes away right after surgery. Then, a few hours, days, or weeks later, the pain returns. This can be related to a number of reasons. The most frequent reason I have seen is that the patient sits, stands, or walks too much and that he or she develops nerve swelling and pain and/or numbness. Usually, the swelling resolves with time as the patient rests and takes it easy. Sometimes, there is muscle spasm in the lower back with increased LBP. This may also resolve with time and the use of a heating pad and muscle relaxant medication. Simple, tolerable low back exercises are recommended.

Weakness after surgery is unusual. What happens is that, once the pain subsides and there is less numbness, the patient can now feel the weakness that was already present before surgery. If there is true weakness after surgery, it will often be related to nerve manipulation. The surgeon will explain the operative findings and work done during surgery. The surgeon will decide if the symptoms after surgery warrant further workup (for example, studies such as an MRI scan). MRI scans obtained right after surgery may be confusing because of the presence of blood from surgery. If the MRI is done several days or weeks later (after surgery), scar tissue may be hard to interpret by the radiologist and the surgeon. One must follow the patient clinically (signs and symptoms) to make a decision on whether or not to reoperate.

Sometimes, there is some bladder discomfort. This could be related to using the Foley catheter during surgery. Usually, this discomfort disappears as time goes by. Notify the physician(s) if symptoms increase in order to begin treatment of a possible urinary infection or prostatitis (male).

Back Brace. Back braces before or after surgery are not routinely recommended because they weaken the lower back muscles and patients may feel more back pain. I recommend a back brace with specific instructions for its use only when a spinal fusion has been performed. The back brace is usually obtained from a local medical supply store. The employee in charge of the braces usually measures the patient, orders a custom-made brace, and instructs the patient on its use. Small adjustments may be done after surgery. It is better to get the back brace before surgery to have it ready following the operation. Soft braces have limited applications. In my opinion, they are of no benefit for stability.

Sex. Most patients are embarrassed to ask about sexual activity. I recommend using common sense and avoid sex for at least the first two to four weeks. After that, avoid awkward positions, and always use common sense. It has been recommended to take the passive position (bottom); however, some people might have back pain while lying on their backs. Probably the best position for sex would be lying on the side.

Special Needs. Sometimes, a hospital bed, high toilet seats, braces, and other special equipment are needed. The insurance company may pay for these, but they will sometimes not cover expenses for this equipment and supplies. Ask your insurance company about coverage for this equipment and medical supplies before surgery if possible.

Allergies. Always inform and remind the physician and all personnel of your allergies to medications, food, or other products (tape). Remind nurse of your allergies before any medication is administered or given to you orally.

Questions. I suggest making a list of all questions the patient or family member may have. I appreciate if the questions are related to issues we have not discussed before surgery. The patient and family members who came to my office before surgery should have read the instructions and information contained on these papers, and they should know which procedure I will be performing.

I will be happy to inform the patient or family members of the findings during surgery, but issues I already discussed extensively before will not be addressed again in the surgical waiting room in order to protect confidentiality.

It is usual that other family members or friends come to the hospital after surgery. They ask questions and bring up issues I have already discussed in detail with the patient before surgery. I would prefer these "new" members ask or discuss those issues with the patient or come to my office for the first postoperative visit so that we may discuss the type of surgery done. I can explain—with the spine model—details and technique of the surgery I performed on the patient.

Paperwork. Bring any paperwork or forms to the physician's office before surgery. If brought to the hospital, they can be misplaced because the physician will be seeing other patients and taking care of medically related problems. Forms can be taken to the office after surgery, but avoid giving papers to the physician when he or she is doing rounds.

Other Issues. Inform your physician (surgeon) of any important details, such as excessive bleeding, pacemakers, recent interventions, dental work, procedures, infections, natural remedies, herbs you are taking, and new medications you started taking after the last visit with the surgeon and before surgery. Notify the surgeon if a new disease was discovered recently that he or she might not be aware of. There are some natural remedies that can cause excessive bleeding and other side effects as well as cause interactions with medications and serious complications. Ask the physician if the plan for surgery is still the same as discussed during the office visit.

Ask any last-minute questions if there are any new issues or concerns before surgery. Arrange for a person to transport you home after surgery. Also, make sure the vehicle is large to be able to lie down on the backseat, recline the front seat, or be lying down or reclined almost all the way down on the way home.

The goals of back surgery are:

- Remove or fix painful spinal conditions
- Help patient improve and get relief from painful symptoms and from neurological deficits (numbness, weakness, sphincter dysfunction, and so forth)
- Decrease the chances for nerve damage
- Improve physical activity and functionality
- Decrease the chances for complications related to inactivity such as blood clot formation in the legs (DVT), heart disease, hypertension, obesity, and diabetes
- Increase self-esteem and decrease the chances for depression and chronic illnesses
- Decrease the chances for drug addiction
- Stabilize the spine when indicated
- Avoid further damage and harm to the patient's spine

Indications for Back Surgery in General

Most textbooks and spine surgeons use well-known and accepted indications for elective low back surgery. Some general indications for surgery may be:

- Persistent LBP and leg pain (incapacitating or disabling)
- Persistent numbness, tingling, or weakness (neurological deficits that may progress)
- Decreased or absent reflexes and other ominous signs found in the exam
- A positive study indicating abnormalities (with clinical correlation)
- Failure to improve with conservative treatment (four to six weeks with some exceptions)

Some Indications for Emergency Spinal Decompressive Surgery

Neurological deficits and/or spinal instability can be indications for emergency surgery.

Some neurological deficits can be:

- Bladder, rectal, or sexual dysfunction with lack of voluntary control (cauda equina syndrome)
- Foot drop or weakness in the leg
- Persistent numbness
- Persistent and severe leg pain or LBP with clear radiological evidence of a spine disorder (HNP, spinal stenosis, spinal hemorrhage, fractures, subluxation, and so forth). These may include radiological studies or other objective documentation. Chronic spinal instability does not necessarily require emergency surgery in all cases (spondylolisthesis, spondylolysis, and so forth).
- Severe LBP is not necessarily an indication for surgery. Severe leg pain might be an indication for urgent surgery, but not necessarily for emergency surgery and only if surgery is objectively warranted (for example, positive MRI scan and/or CT scan and neurological deficits or impairment).

Cases with partial cauda equina are more common than previously thought. Recent studies revealed that partial cauda equina was more common than detected on a routine history and exam.

Severe pain should be considered as an emergency. However, many health insurance companies do not consider pain as an emergency. There are cases of patients with severe pain in which neither elective nor emergency surgery applies. Patients with severe LBP and/or leg pain do not necessarily require emergency surgery, but they can neither wait several days or weeks for surgery. Pain can be severe and incapacitating. These patients typically go to an emergency room, are treated with painkillers, and then released to their primary care physician. Severe pain does not warrant surgery without clinical and radiological correlation. However, patients sometimes need hospitalization for pain management.

Surgery should be indicated based on both clinical and radiological evidence of a surgical condition. However, there are cases in which surgery is strongly considered based on radiological studies, even on patients with mild symptoms because they may be at a risk for potential complications if surgery is not done in a timely manner. On the other hand, there are patients whose symptoms appear to be more elaborate when trying to correlate radiological studies. We have to remember there is no one hundred percent test or study that will accurately show the cause of pain. I have done surgery on patients who had a "benign" MRI scan or it showed only mild abnormalities. However, during surgery, I encountered variants and undetected presurgical findings, such as small fragments of disc lodged or wedged in the lateral recess or in the foramen, vascular variants with large veins pressing the nerves, ligamentum flavum in the lateral recess trapping the nerves, double or conjoined nerve root, and so forth. These abnormalities may not be detected before surgery. We do have to be cautious though with the patient that exaggerates symptoms.

The MRI scan plays a significant role in the decision-making process. Recent publications indicate that people with a disc herniation and a "free fragment" can be treated conservatively. Once again, it all depends on the level of herniation in the spine. For instance, the L4-5 level is narrower than L5-S1, and the L4-5 spinal canal is less tolerant of occupying masses of disc herniation or free fragments. Other issues are also considered, such as the possibility of neurological deficits, severe leg pain, medical status, and size of the person. Surgeons try to avoid surgery as much as possible when there are conservative or semiconservative ways of treating a patient with LBP.

There are situations in which surgery may be controversial. Surgeons may have different opinions for indicating surgery, depending on their experience, medical education, and training in a specialty. Neurosurgeons and orthopedic surgeons are currently doing spine surgery. There might be a subtle difference of opinions between neurosurgeons and orthopedic surgeons when recommending certain surgical techniques.

What does low back surgery involve? How many types of surgery exist? How do I know which surgery I need? When is the best time for surgery? What is the best technique in spine surgery? Patients ask me these questions frequently.

The answer is that there is no perfect spine surgery. However, we, as surgeons, should do the surgery that most likely will benefit the patient. Every surgical technique is different for each patient with the same spinal condition. The surgical technique chosen is directly related to the patient's age, constitution, size, needs, physical demands, as well as social and cultural demands. For instance, an older person with a herniated disc may not be a candidate for decompression and spinal fusion, whereas a young person who does heavy work may need a more aggressive approach with decompression and maybe even a spinal fusion. One of the rules of surgery is not to cause more pain or harm to the patient. We do not want to endanger the patient's life when there are other options for treatment with less risk.

Work demands, psychological status, and motivation are also important when choosing one surgery over others. It has been concluded that patients suffering from depression or a compulsive disorder may not be good surgical candidates. Aggressive surgeries with spinal fusion carry a relatively high incidence of complications.

There is common consensus when treating certain spinal conditions, particularly with surgery. Most surgeons will agree a patient with spondylolisthesis (dislocation or slippage of one vertebra over another) could represent an indication for a spinal fusion surgery if instability is demonstrated or suspected. Fracture and dislocation due to trauma or cancer are also specific indications for a spinal fusion.

The gray and controversial area is on patients with a small slippage (grade I or II). I tend not to recommend an aggressive spinal fusion with hardware to the elderly with medical problems and a small slippage. The young, working person may benefit from a spinal fusion (there are several types of spinal fusion techniques) if there is a grade II or evidence of instability of the spine along with symptoms that match the radiological studies.

Different people may have the same condition but they may be treated differently after considering all circumstances. Some factors may alter the outcome of surgery. For instance, the smoker, the obese, the diabetic, the elderly, the depressed, the terminally ill, and other patients may not recuperate very well after surgery. Social and cultural issues must also be considered when doing back surgery.

Surgery should not be based solely on a radiological study, on a person's demands, or on one single factor. All factors and circumstances have to be balanced to reach the best decision for surgery on a patient.

The surgeon may recommend surgery, but the patient should also participate in the decision-making process. The patient makes the decision of surgery with the information the physician gives. However, the surgeon should elect the surgical technique for the particular patient he or she is treating. The chosen surgical technique, complications, and recovery time should be clearly explained to the patient.

What Are the Indications for Spine Surgery with Spinal Instrumentation (Fusion)?

These are some specific indications for using hardware or spinal instrumentation:

- Spinal fractures with spinal instability (demonstrated with radiological studies)
- Spinal instability related to degenerative processes
- Spinal instability after a surgical procedure (iatrogenic)
- Failed back surgery (relative indication for instrumentation)
- "Salvage surgery" (surgery that follows a first fusion operation in which there was a complication such as breakage of screws, rods, cages, or plates)
- Instability related to destructive bone and joint lesions such as in the case of spinal tumor
- Deformities of the spine with symptoms and radiological evidence of instability
- End plate abnormalities with erosion and/or bone destruction that can be related to a number of causes (for example, infection, tumor, trauma, genetic, and congenital)

"Discogenic Disc Disease" (also called Degenerative Disc Disease or DDD) is a disorder still under research in which some clinicians and researchers believe that some patients have LBP and leg pain related to the degenerative disc. DDD is not necessarily the cause of "discogenic pain." DDD can be seen in an MRI scan of normal people (without LBP). When a patient has DDD by MRI scan, some clinicians perform a discogram to try to differentiate the painful DDD from the painless. I consider a discogram or discography study unreliable if surgery is based only on scattered clinical information and radiological data.

Indications for spinal instrumentation can be a controversial matter. Many patients underwent surgeries for "Discogenic Disc Disease" or for degenerative disc disease (DDD) in the 1990s. Many of these patients represent the vast majority crowding pain clinics now.

A different group of patients is those who have endplate erosion. These patients may, at the same time, represent three different types or subgroups: vertebral end plate edema, replacement of bone marrow by fat, and osteosclerosis. In these cases, the flat surface of the vertebral body (superior or inferior) erodes. There can be several causes of these changes such as genetic, congenital, trauma, infection, and tumor-related. These end plate abnormalities are also called "internal or vertical disc rupture or herniation." Some of these patients may represent surgical candidates for fusion surgery with hardware.

Spine surgeons learned to be more cautious and gained more respect for these operations. Currently, spine surgeons are less aggressive than in the 1990s. Less spinal instrumentation surgeries are carried out.

Another area of controversy is the indication for a spinal fusion after "failed" disc surgery. There seems to be common consensus in the indications for a spinal fusion after a third operation for disc herniation. But, again, there are exceptions, and one must be cautious and wonder why the first two operations "failed."

Contraindications for Back Surgery

These are some absolute contraindications for elective back surgery:

- No clinical (on the medical history and exam) or diagnostic (studies) evidence of a condition that explains the patient's symptoms. Surgery should be carried out only if within reasonable medical and surgical probabilities and the possibility there is a greater chance of improvement with surgery. Otherwise, surgery should not be undertaken.

- Debilitating medical conditions (AIDS, cancer, and immunosuppressed patients)

- Infection processes (systemic)

- Coagulopathies or blood disease patients on certain medications (aspirin, coumadin, and other blood thinners)

- Systemic medical conditions such as heart, lung, or renal disease. These patients must be medically optimized for surgery, and there will be cases in which surgery is contraindicated because of the high risk for complications and death.

- Surgery against the patient's consent

- Mental disease that may endanger postoperative outcome. Depressed patients do not fare well. Some spine surgeons do not perform back surgery on a certain patient unless the patient has been first evaluated by a psychiatrist and/or a psychologist. When malingering or secondary gain is suspected, an MMPI or other psychological tests may be needed. If the patient shows symptoms and signs of magnification, some surgeons do not perform surgery on these patients even if there are abnormalities on the radiological studies.
- Patients with current diseases such as pneumonia, severe liver disease, deep venous thrombosis, and pulmonary embolus or recent heart attack or high risk of heart complications (American Heart Association classification)
- Osteoporosis may be contraindications for certain types of spinal fusion.

Other relative contraindications for back surgery include:

- Patients with lung, heart, liver or renal disease, diabetes, gout, or some other systemic disease. The patient will have to be optimized (cleared) by the respective specialist.
- Osteoporosis
- Underlying bone and joint disease
- Certain mental conditions
- Obesity. Some surgeons will not do surgery on overweight patients until they lose weight. The truth is that most patients will not lose weight because they are in pain and cannot exercise. They are sedentary.
- Smokers
- Alcoholism
- Drug addiction
- AIDS, hepatitis, and other immunodeficiency and debilitating conditions
- Secondary gain
- Age is not necessarily a contraindication for surgery. Several factors have to be considered, however, because we cannot deny that elderly patients are more prone to develop certain complications. Pain is universal, regardless of age, and affects all groups of people. A physician should not underestimate the elderly. They also have severe pain, and it is not fair that patients suffer only because they are "too old." Physicians sometimes have the concept that some patients are too old for surgery or cer-

tain treatments. Surgery is beneficial to the patient in some cases. There are cultures such as the Hispanic in which they tend to believe the elderly should not have any kind of surgery because they are "too old for surgery." They believe the elderly "do not have many years to live" and surgery could be a fatal risk. It is difficult to convince them otherwise.

Although age is not necessarily a contraindication for surgery (as I stated before), surgeons should weigh the benefits of surgery and complications on an elderly patient. One must consider special situations such as patients with osteoporosis, underlying bone or joint disease, cancer, rheumatoid arthritis, and so forth. Patients with some medical conditions should undergo certain studies before surgery. For instance, a patient with rheumatoid arthritis may need a neck X-ray prior to surgery to rule out cervical dislocation, which is more common in patients with rheumatoid arthritis. One, as a surgeon, must consider several factors when doing surgery on a patient. Alcoholism, smoking, morbid obesity, and other habits may not be a contraindication for surgery, but it is strongly recommended to control these habits before surgery.

How do surgeons determine the good and poor candidates for surgery?

Several factors are used to consider good or bad surgical candidates. Candidates for back surgery include:

- Patients motivated to improve and have an active, productive life
- Patients who demonstrate commitment and compliance with the surgeon's recommendations
- Patients who have a condition in which clinical and radiological data are consistent
- Patients with no underlying bone or joint condition
- No history of smoking, obesity, or other medical systemic disease

Challenge patients include:

- Malingerers with a true surgical condition
- Obese patients
- Smokers, alcoholics, or drug users
- Patients with chronic back pain
- Pain related to underlying medical conditions, such as diabetes, heart disease, lung disease, and so forth

- Patients with bone and joint disorders (for example, rheumatoid arthritis and other joint progressive disease)
- Patients with depression and other mental conditions
- Patients with secondary gain (litigious patients, patients under workers' compensation, and so forth)
- Noncompliant patients
- Patients with previous back surgery (or surgeries)
- Elderly patients

What Do We Mean When We Talk of "Back Surgery"?

People refer to "back surgery" as if all back surgeries are the same. I would like to explain some of the current surgical techniques the surgeon has to consider. Although the surgeon should involve the patient in the decision-making process for surgery, the surgeon should recommend one technique over another. But, he or she should explain the reasoning behind his or her decision.

Surgical Techniques for the Lower Back

There are at least four primary surgical procedures and variants for the lower back:

1. Laminectomy (decompressive)

   a) Laminectomy + fusion

2. Disc excision (diskectomy or discectomy), also decompression of the nerve roots

   a) Discectomy + fusion

   b) Laminectomy + discectomy

   c) Laminectomy + discectomy + fusion (with or without hardware)

   d) Disc excision and disc replacement

3. Corrective surgery for spinal deformities, fractures, and dislocations

4. Minimally invasive procedures

These are some of the common surgical techniques utilized for low back surgery:

- Standard posterior discectomy (and anterior discectomy)
- Microdiskectomy (posterior)

- Endoscopic discectomy or percutaneous discectomy (with or without laser)
- Nucleoplasty
- Thermal disc treatment of the DDD
- Laminectomy, hemilaminectomy, laminotomy, foraminotomy, partial medial facetectomy
- Laminoplasty
- Artificial disc replacement
- Spinal fusion (with and without hardware and with bone fusion). The bone utilized can be:
  - Allograft
  - Autologous bone or autograft
  - Combination of both
  - Artificial (ceramic) graft

There are combinations of the above procedures as well as variants for a diskectomy. It can be microdiskectomy, endoscopic discectomy (with or without laser), IDET, injection of the disc (papain), and so forth. The laminectomy is a standard procedure. For a fusion, there are several variants, techniques, and companies that design different hardware (plates, screws, rods, and cages). There are newer techniques for treating herniated discs, such as a transforaminal discectomy, which is a different anatomical approach to the disc; endoscopy with or without laser discectomy; and fusion with plates, rods, screws, and, most recently, artificial discs.

Spinal Fusion. Usually, a spinal fusion (with or without instrumentation) is performed after some kind of decompression of the spinal cord and/or nerves. A spinal fusion can be done with or without metal. Bone is usually used on either one. There can be bone taken from the patient having surgery (autologous bone) or from a cadaver (allograft). There is artificial bone-like material, such as ceramic, that is also used instead of true bone. Metal cages are also used.

The spinal fusion surgical techniques can be:

- Bone fusion alone with no spinal instrumentation
  - Facet joint fusion (arthrodesis)
  - Transverse process technique
  - Intervertebral fusion (bone or metal cage), anterior or posterior
- Spinal instrumentation with bone fusion

- Endoscopic spinal fusion (minimally invasive spine surgery)

Spinal instrumentation and bone fusion can be:

- Anterior
- Posterior
- Lateral
- Combined

Type of hardware used for spinal instrumentation fusion:

- Screws (pedicle, lateral mass, transverse process, facet screws, and so forth)
- Hooks
- Rods
- Cable and wire
- Plates
- Interbody cages
- Disc replacement

Types of instrumentation spinal fusion include:

- CD (Cotrel-Dubousset)
- Kaneda
- Harrington
- Luque
- BAK Lumbar interbody fusion
- TSRH
- Isola
- PLIF (posterior lateral interbody fusion)
- Songer Cable, soft wire
- ALPS (anterior locking plate lab)
- CASP (Contour Anterior Spinal Plate lab)
- Z Plate
- Modular Spine Rod Linkage System
- Ray Cage, BAK, and other types of "cages" (Bone, Ceramic, Carbon Fiber)
- PLIF and cage combined

- Interlaminar wires and cables
- Facet and spinous process screws and wiring (with or without involvement of the transverse process)
- Laminoplasty with or without fusion

Some of the above fusion techniques have been abandoned or substituted for more current techniques considered to be safer and less complex.

A couple of techniques have been developed recently for the patient with vertebral collapsing (particularly for the patient with osteoporosis): vertebroplasty and kyphoplasty. I have already discussed these techniques in the section of semiconservative treatment of the patient with LBP.

These are some comments I would like to make in reference to the treatment of a patient with LBP:

Microdiscectomy (Microdiskectomy). Although it is the procedure of choice by several spine surgeons, the success rate has been underrated. The complications rate is low (one to seven percent depending on the series and studies). The success rate used to be reported as high as ninety percent in some series, but, most recently, studies have published an initial success rate (first weeks after surgery) as high as ninety percent, but the success rate decreased over time to about seventy-five percent after one to two years. There are several reasons for this decline, such as further spinal deterioration as part of the aging process, obesity, smoking, poor body biomechanics, reinjury, scar tissue formation, and so forth. However, this is the surgical technique of choice by most spine surgeons for a patient with a disc herniation.

Laser Surgery. Spinal fusion or some other surgical technique with the use of lasers or with the use of fancy technology not necessarily increases the operative success rate. On the contrary, it has been seen in some studies that, when using these techniques, some patients require another surgery at another time. I am not aware that surgeons use the laser for open surgery. There is the assumption by patients—and sometimes even by primary physicians—that the patient has an increased success rate when compared with a conventional microdiscectomy at a local hospital because laser surgery is used. This assumption is a misconception.

Fusion Surgery. One should be aware that spinal fusion surgery is more expensive and that surgeons get compensated more than for a "simple" surgery. Because there are many different companies with different hardware equipment, there may not be consistent, prospective, randomized studies of more than ten years old and with specific clinical data studies to favor one technique or piece of equipment over another. However, some techniques and equipment have been discontinued because of the high incidence of complications and poor outcome on patients.

As a patient, one must remember that, as medicine evolves, patients still fall under the "guinea pig studies." For a scientific study to be valid, it must include a large population of patients with exactly the same medical condition (spine) and same body constitution. The study must include other factors as a cause of LBP, such as obesity, smoking, psychological personality, and so forth. Long-term (five to ten years), double-blinded studies are needed to determine with more accuracy more realistic statistical results.

- When speaking of surgery, there is no "easy" or "simple" surgery; however, there are surgical techniques that, because of the nature of the operation, are more complex to perform. Thus, the complication rate increases.

- Very few patients indeed require an aggressive operation with hardware. This may be the reason why patients may require more than one surgery or for the increasing proliferation of "pain clinics."

Successful Surgery. One must be cautious when considering "success rate." One consideration is success rate when speaking of fusion success rate; another issue is the patient's success rate. They do not go hand in hand. A patient may have an excellent postoperative X-ray showing a very good fusion site, but the patient may be having the same pain as before surgery or even more pain. This would be considered as a successful fusion operation but unsuccessful patient outcome.

One must be cautious, as a surgeon, when reporting in our medical reports, "The patient presents with a very successful fusion." Furthermore, one may have a poor fusion success rate with an X-ray that shows that the fusion is not "taking." There may be pseudoarthrosis or some other complication seen on the X-rays, but the patient may be improving. This will be a successful surgery with a patient who has improved (which is the goal and the more important issue) and an unsuccessful fusion. Many times, these patients that present with an "unsuccessful" postoperative X-ray are left alone with no more operations if—clinically speaking—the patient is improving. We do not treat X-rays; we treat patients!

Other techniques used in surgery to augment the success rate.

- Efforts are made to prevent the formation of scar tissue after back surgery. Different techniques have been attempted, such as the use of free fat (fat taken from under the patient's skin) as well as different substances and gels (including pieces of plastic-like materials). No technique has proven to be one hundred percent effective to this date.

- There is also the use of "bone stimulators." They are electricity-based devices used in some occasions to increase the chance for a bone fusion.

- Newer techniques in surgery are under development. These techniques are designed to increase the chances for a successful operation.

- Stimulators of bone formation come in different presentations and are usually used as a mixed matrix mixed with blood from the same patient having surgery.

- There is the use of bone graft already prepared for implantation in the spine (measured and shaped). There are different types of bone grafts used for spinal fusion surgery, including "autologous" bone grafts (from the same patient having surgery) and allograft (bone from cadaver, already prepared and sterilized). There are also ceramic, metal (titanium), and carbon-based implants (cages). These grafts are used mostly for spinal fusion. They have been used to increase the bone fusion rate and to keep anatomical alignment.

- New implants such as "artificial disc" have been used in Europe for a few years. These new techniques and implants for spine surgery are still under FDA scrutiny for possible approval for use in the United States.

- A newer technique used in spine surgery is called "spinal navigation." Spinal navigation is based on image-guided surgical technology designed to improve spatial anatomical 3-D orientation of the unseen anatomical structures during surgery (unexposed anatomy during surgery) for the surgeon during certain cases of complex spinal surgery.

Spinal navigation also decreases exposure of the patient, the surgeon, and the operating team to radiation during the obtaining of intraoperative X-rays. Currently, some spine surgeons use conventional X-rays and fluoroscopy (dynamic, real-time radiographs) for the placement of hardware, such as screws, plates, cages, and other devices, into the spine.

Spinal navigation is not necessarily a new concept. Spinal navigation derived from the use of stereotactic intracranial surgery that has been used for several years. Spinal navigation establishes a correlation between the intraoperative anatomy and a preoperative CT scan data. There are different navigational systems, but most of them rely on a reference point or a frame of reference (a fixation device that is applied to certain anatomical structure(s) during spine surgery). Coordinates are calculated through a computerized system.

Not all spine centers are equipped with this technology, and this technology is not essential for a surgeon to perform spine surgery. This technology is mostly used for complex spine cases such as the placement of screws, plates, rods, cages, and other devices in the spine.

At this time, I would like to make some comments related to the use and implant of artificial disc surgery.

The use of *artificial disc surgery* has been carried out in Europe for some time. Comparative studies of fusion and disc replacement have taken place in Europe. BAK is one of the operations compared with disc replacement. The outcome and success rate are very similar. The complication rate is also similar. There is possibly a little better outcome in the patients with disc replacement.

The rational of disc replacement and BAK (fusion) is completely different—biomechanically speaking. In spinal fusion (BAK), two vertebral bodies are fused and immobilized. In disc replacement, the principle is the opposite. Keep the disc segment mobile, as in the normal spine. The advantages of disc replacement are that the disc takes the anatomical position of the normal disc, and it allows the spine to move close to the normal spine. The disadvantage is that usually disc replacement is indicated for only one segment (L4-5 or L5-S1) and only for the L4-5 and L5-S1 levels, but not for higher levels. Therefore, patients with multiple disc disease cannot have this procedure done.

The surgeon performing disc replacement should be skillful because this operation requires a great deal of precision. Patients for disc replacement have to be carefully selected. Another disadvantage of disc replacement is that surgery is performed through the front part of the spine (retroperitoneal or transperitoneal). It requires a general surgeon to expose the anterior portion of the spine. Serious complications can occur with these operations related to the abdominal and pelvic organs, nerves, and large blood vessels.

Spinal surgeons are more familiar with spinal posterior or posterior-lateral fusion surgery. They are less familiar, however, with anterior operations (that require a general surgeon).

What are the indications for another surgery? Do they work? These are some of the common questions patients ask me when they already had surgery and have been recommended to have another operation.

These are some indications for further (after a first operation) surgery can be (but are not limited to):

- Retained fragment of a disc herniation
- Operation at the wrong level of the spine
- Recurrent disc herniation

- Infection
- Complications from hardware if spinal instrumentations have been used, such as breakage of hardware screws, rods, and pins. Screw dislodgment, infections, and contamination of the hardware.
- Pseudoarthrosis (lack of bone fusion). The fusion site does not "take," and there is mobility and pain with this condition.
- Increased deterioration of the spine
- Another spinal level developing disc herniation, stenosis, or simply further deterioration
- Incomplete decompression of the spine
- Prior instability not detected before the first surgery or creation of spinal instability during surgery by removing too much bone or removing the joints and the stabilizing elements of the spine
- Inadvertent fractures and iatrogenic injuries (dura tears, arachnoid cyst, synovial cyst, and so forth)

Most surgeons do not recommend surgery for scar tissue removal because another surgery guarantees further scar tissue formation (probably more than after the first surgery). Some surgeons are talked into doing another surgery only for the patient's secondary gain, either maliciously or unintentionally (psychological conflicts). Whether or not another surgery will work depends on several factors, such as indications for the first operation(s), type of surgery performed, age of the person, motivation for work, poor body mechanics and ergonomics, and so forth. The use of radiation and even gamma knife is under investigation for the treatment of pain related to scar tissue around the nerves (and arachnoiditis).

These are some illustrations of frames used in back surgery:

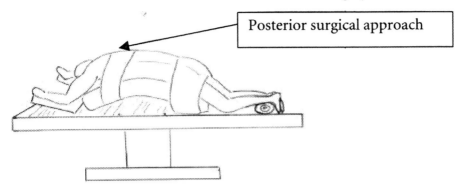

Posterior surgical approach

This is one of the most common frames and positions used for back surgery.

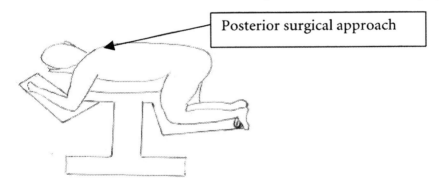

Posterior surgical approach

There are different frames used for back surgery.

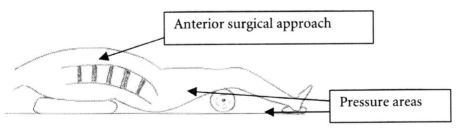

Anterior surgical approach

Pressure areas

These drawings represent different positions utilized during spine surgery. During surgery, one must be cautious with the pressure areas of the body, including the eyes. (Blindness has occurred because of prolonged pressure of the eyes during surgery.) Peripheral nerves can also be compressed during surgery.

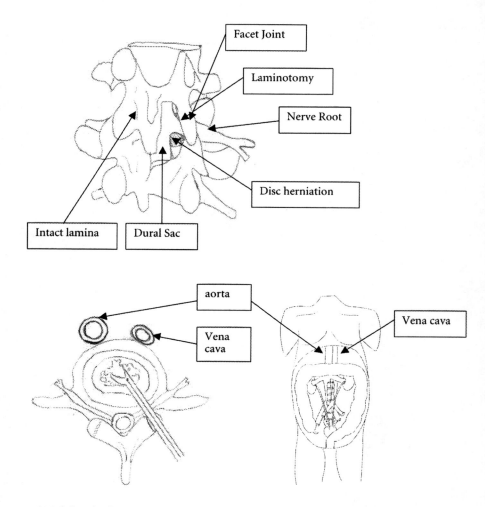

Axial (top) view.

During a discectomy, a grasping instrument or forceps is used to remove the disc herniation. Care must be taken to avoid inserting the instrument too deep because intra-abdominal organs and the great vessels can be damaged with devastating consequences.

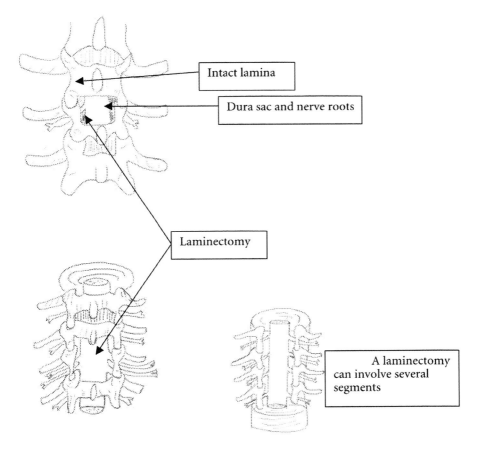

Intact lamina

Dura sac and nerve roots

Laminectomy

A laminectomy can involve several segments

Posterior view of the spine.

Laminectomy is one of the most frequent procedures performed in the spine to relieve pressure off the nerves and the spinal cord. Care must be taken to avoid taking excessive bone that could lead to instability of the spine.

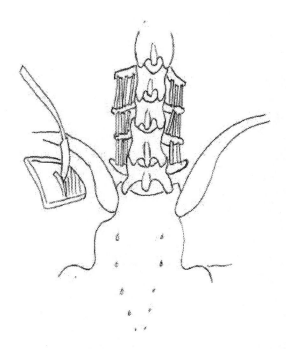

A spinal fusion may involve the placement of bone graft (usually taken out of the iliac bone) over the decorticated vertebrae. This is called "bone fusion." The bone fusion can involve the facet joints or the facet joints and the transverse processes. No hardware is used in a bone fusion.

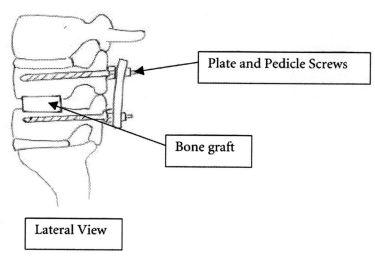

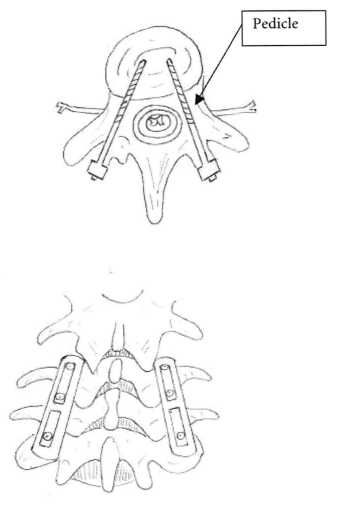

Pedicle

Axial and posterior views of the spine.

A posterior spinal fusion with instrumentation or hardware is shown above. Bone graft (bone chips) is scattered around the hardware. Bone graft can be obtained from a bone bank (cadaver).

CHAPTER 5

Surgical Complications

Who Talks of Complications in Surgery?

Most surgeons will generally tell patients some of the most frequent complications that could result after surgery. Surgical complications can occur during and after an operation (intraoperative and postoperative respectively). They can manifest immediately, or they can appear later on. Immediate complications may be recognized, repaired, or fixed at that time with no subsequent repercussions or neurological deficits. They may develop following surgery, even after repairing the complication during the same operation. There can also be complications that can develop if surgery is not performed timely.

There is a difference in the complication rate of patients who have a spinal instrumentation operation and the ones who do not. In general, the complication rate for patients who undergo surgery without a spinal fusion with instrumentation is around three to six percent. The complications are usually related to infection, bleeding, dura tear, nerve damage, spinal instability, scar tissue, recurrent disc herniation, recurrent pain, or pseudoarthrosis (partial bone fusion). The complication rate on patients who had a decompressive procedure and a spinal fusion with hardware (in general) can be as high as fifteen or twenty percent. There are studies that mention a thirty-five percent complication rate after spinal instrumentation fusion surgery. The type and rate of complications depend on the procedure that was used; the patient's condition; physical fitness; or preoperative factors, such as smoking, obesity, poor body posture (mechanics), poor compliance, and underlying bone and joint disease. There are surgeons who claim to have a very low complication rate even when using hardware for a spinal fusion. One must be skeptical when data can be manipulated either way.

In general, the complication rate of surgery for the lower back with and without hardware varies significantly, sometimes with a ten to fifteen percent higher rate for patients with hardware.

Ironically, it has been proven, most recently, that certain patients (with spondylolisthesis grade I and even II) who underwent a bone fusion surgery without instrumentation fare better than the ones with hardware. Spine surgeons performed bone fusion surgery alone (without hardware) about thirty to forty years ago.

What Kind of Surgical Complications Are We Talking About?

There can be complications directly related and others not directly related to a certain procedure. There are the complications that can occur on both groups of patient with a spinal fusion (with and without hardware).

These are some of the complications in general related to spine surgery with and without hardware:

- Infection
- Hemorrhage
- Increased instability (and facet joint injury with pain and instability)
- Intra-abdominal organ injury (arterial of venous, ureter or kidney injury, intestinal and other organ injury)
- Spinal fluid leak related to a dura tear or nerve damage (with or without neurological deficits). There is a complication related to a dura tear that is called pseudomeningocele, or accumulation of spinal fluid under the skin. (In some cases, another surgery is needed to repair it.) Synovial and pseudosynovial cyst can occur after surgery.
- Wrong level of surgery
- Surgical materials (sponge) inadvertently left inside the wound
- Scar tissue formation (exuberant) and recurrent or persistent pain
- Recurrent stenosis and/or disc herniation
- Pseudoarthrosis (with or without clinical manifestations)
- Incomplete decompression
- Retained (missed) disc fragment (in the case of a discectomy)
- Skin reaction to sutures, tape, and hardware
- Cosmetic deformity (bad scar)
- Reflex Sympathetic Dystrophy (RSD) or Complex Regional Pain Syndrome (CRPS) type I

- Compressive neuropathies related to the position during surgery
- Genital injury for prolonged compression during surgery
- Skin irritation and blistering from the operating frame used
- Joint pain after surgery, also related to inadequate padding and joint position during surgery (knee, elbow, shoulder, and so forth)
- Complications related to a bone graft itself or to the donor site if a bone fusion takes place in surgery (these complications are addressed below)
- Subdural cranial or spinal hematoma
- Unusual complications related to spine surgery
- Prominent hardware irritating the soft tissues and skin
- Other

The complications listed below are mostly related to the use of hardware:

- Increased pain (back and/or leg pain) with poor outcomes ("failed back surgery")
- Increased infection rate
- Increased risk for hemorrhage
- Increased postoperative pain (longer incision, more extensive soft tissue destruction and exposure)
- Increased rehabilitation (not always)
- More chances for using narcotic pain medication and drug addiction if there is more postoperative pain
- More chances for depression and other adverse psychological impact of a failed surgery. (This complication also has other social and economical repercussions.)
- Pseudoarthrosis and increased pain
- Synovial and pseudosynovial cyst formation
- The need for another surgery to correct complications of previous surgery
- Impotence and bladder dysfunction if an anterior approach has been used (retrograde ejaculation)
- Reflex Sympathetic Dystrophy (RSD). (It may be more likely than on back surgery without hardware.)
- Further deterioration of the spine at the same operated level or at levels above and below. (Further surgery may be required.)

- Increased disability
- Increased instability and deformity
- Complications directly related to the hardware:
- Breakage of the screws, cages, rods, or plates
- Penetration of metal into the bone and spontaneous screw back out
- Fractures caused by the hardware
- Body rejection to foreign body (metal)
- Painful protrusion of hardware under the skin
- Migration of hardware that can result in devastating complications, such as nerve damage, increased LBP or leg pain, and even paralysis. There can be intra-abdominal organ and vascular injury. (This complication can be fatal.)

- Others
  Complications of bone graft can be (but are not limited to):
- Allograft
  - The allograft can collapse or break.
  - The allograft can carry bacterial or viral infections, fungus, HIV, as well as hepatitis B and C. (The chances of contracting HIV are 1 in 49,000 cases; for hepatitis B, it's 1 in 6,300 cases. For hepatitis C, which is deadly after several years, the frequency is about 1 in 2,500, but the infection window for hepatitis C is longer, and it may be undetected in some cases.)
  - There can be rejection of the foreign bone by the patient undergoing surgery.
- Autograft
  The complications of autograft related to the bone donor site can be:
  - Pain
  - Nerve damage (nerves in the area of the incision)
  - Intra-abdominal or pelvic organ injury
  - Cosmetic deformity
  - Pelvic bone (iliac or sacrum) fractures
  - Vascular injury
- Ceramic or other material bone-like grafts
  - Rejection

- Infection
- Migration
- Systemic reactions

The three types of grafts can migrate posteriorly and pinch nerves and even the spinal cord. They can migrate anteriorly and compromise intra-abdominal or pelvic organs. Grafts can fracture the vertebrae, sinking into the bone (subsidence) with resulting severe pain, instability, pseudoarthrosis (non-fusion), and/or neurological impairment.

There can be other systemic complications not directly related to surgery that may affect other organs in the body. These systemic complications can occur on patients who undergo back surgery with and without hardware.

- Deep venous thrombosis (DVT). It can be more common on patients who have hardware surgery.
- Pulmonary embolism (serious complication that may result in death). It is also more frequent on patients who had spinal instrumentation surgery.
- Peptic ulcer and bleeding (probably the same complication rate on both groups)
- Constipation and intestinal perforation in severe cases. (It is more likely on patients with hardware.)
- Heart attack, lung disease (pneumonia, exacerbation of emphysema, asthma). These complications can be the same in both groups; however, if there has been significant blood loss, there are more chances for heart disease. There is also a risk of stroke.
- Complications related to diabetes (hypo- or hyperglycemia). The same rate probably applies for both groups.
- Bladder infections and/or prostate exacerbation of a previous condition (probably the same complication rate for both groups)
- Medication and anesthesia-related
- In some cases, one must check for cervical stability and degree of spondylosis. A patient with cervical spinal stenosis and/or instability may have catastrophic complications after low back surgery that can result in paralysis from the neck down (quadriplegia). Surgeons must be especially cautious with patients who have a previous history of neck surgery, injuries (fracture and subluxation), and underlying diseases such as rheumatoid arthritis that are sometimes associated with cervical instability.
- Others

Surgeons typically inform patients of the most frequent complications that may occur during or after surgery.

There are patients who tell me: "Doc, just do whatever you think needs to be done. You are the doctor, you are the specialist, and I trust you; I do not want to know anything about it." I still emphasize and clarify to the patient what the most common surgical complications are.

By no means, the complications I mentioned above are to scare patients from having back surgery. I think patients should be entitled to at least know that some operations have a higher risk of complications. Therefore, a more cautious and conscientious decision is made for surgery by the surgeon and patient. The reason for selecting certain types of surgery is very important.

Complications of Semiconservative Treatment. There is a subset of complications related to minimally invasive procedures and the ones related to semiconservative treatment (invasive procedures).

Some of the complications resulting from minimally invasive procedures can be related to the use of needles, probes, and reactions to the medications and materials used for the procedures. Some of these complications can be fatal. Some of these complications can be:

- Infection
- Hemorrhage
- Intra-abdominal, intrathoracic, or pelvic organ injury
- Disc herniation (related to the performance of a discography)
- Neurological impairment secondary to nerve or spinal cord injury
- Fracture, collapsing of the vertebras
- Pain
- Scar tissue formation and secondary complications
- Medications-related complications (side effects)

There are complications related to the use of certain device implants such as morphine pump, spinal stimulator, and others. These complications can be:

- Device dislodgments or migration (and disconnecting problems)
- Malfunction of the device
- Body rejection to the material of the device
- Side effects related to the medications dispensed with these devices
- Hemorrhage
- Infections

- CSF leak (meningitis in some cases)
- Spinal stroke
- Respiratory depression (and even death)
- Neurological deficits and impairment that can be temporary or permanent (paralysis)

Complications Related to Conservative Treatment. These complications are frequently related to constant pressure over the nerves (by a disc herniation, a tight ligament, or bone encroachment) and to inactivity. Some of these complications can be:

- Nerve damage that can be permanent or temporary (with subsequent paralysis, pain, numbness, and sphincter dysfunction)
- Inactivity and subsequent conditions associated are heart disease, diabetes, obesity, depression, and deep venous thrombosis (DVT).
- Further spinal deterioration with worsening of the symptoms

"Failed Back Surgery/Disastrous Back Surgery." Surgeons use the terms "failed back surgery" for patients who had back surgery and continued to have LBP and/or leg pain after several months of surgery. The term "disastrous back surgery" refers to the patient who not only did not improve after surgery, but got worse related to an adverse outcome after surgery.

These are some of the most frequent causes of persistent LBP and/or leg pain after surgery:

- Chronic LBP
- Chronic depression and other psychological issues including secondary gain
- Surgery performed at the wrong level of the spine
- Incomplete surgery
- Aggressive surgery (long incision, extensive muscle trauma, and excessive bone removal)
- Facet joint invasion or transgression
- Scar tissue formation (and exuberant scar tissue formation)
- Infection
- Inaccurate diagnosis
- Overlapping musculoskeletal conditions (for instance, spinal stenosis and osteoporosis)

- Overlapping systemic disorders, such as diabetic sciatica, rheumatoid arthritis, medication-related pain (anticholesterol, anticancer, and other drugs)

- Progressive, underlying musculoskeletal and joint disease (for example, rheumatoid arthritis, osteoarthritis, osteoporosis)

- Compliance issues (reaggravation of back conditions)

- Recurrent disc herniation and other recurrent spinal disorders

- Iatrogenic, physician-caused pain with surgery (instability, joint invasion, synovial or pseudosynovial cyst, fracture, and so forth). Some kinds of conservative treatments, spinal manipulations, injections, and so forth may not be the best procedure for a particular patient.

- Legal issues (workers' compensation, motor vehicle accident, and so forth)

- Normal expected aging and further spinal and bone deterioration

- Pseudoarthrosis is a term used by physicians to refer to the lack of bone fusion when a spinal "fusion" surgery has been performed. The bone does not fuse or unite, and there is partial motion of the joints or bone to be fused. These conditions can cause chronic pain. However, not all patients who develop "pseudoarthrosis" have pain, and not all the patients who show an "excellent" bone fusion on X-rays are pain-free.

- Poor posture and awkward positions when standing and walking, resulting in unbalanced joint structures, such as feet, ankles, knees, hips, pelvis, and spine

How about the kind of back surgery to be performed? This is also a contributing factor in the complex equation of LBP + Diagnosis + Treatment + Outcome.

Sometimes, a poor outcome with persistent LBP and/or leg pain can cause anxiety and frustration to be replaced by anger. The surgeon should explain these possible consequences before surgery. In fact, most surgeons will say there is no one hundred percent guarantee of success with surgery. Others may say there is a "50-50" success rate, which I think is unfair. If there has been a thorough preoperative evaluation, the most appropriate surgery is selected, and good postoperative care is taken, the patient should improve the odds. That is why surgery is an important event, and it deserves careful planning.

Controversies in Spine Surgery

The following statements can be debatable and controversial:

- Not all individuals with LBP have the same spinal condition.
- Not all people with LBP should be treated the same way.
- Age, medical fitness and condition, habits (smoking, overweight, and so forth), psychological problems, and litigation are factors that may contribute to the decision-making process of the physician on treatment of the lower back pain patient.
- Duration of symptoms is also very controversial and misleading. A patient with a herniated disc and a free fragment may be at risk of having permanent nerve damage if surgery is delayed six to twelve weeks as typically recommended (waiting to spontaneously heal with conservative treatment). Conversely, patients that have been in pain for a long time not necessarily require surgery. Patients should be treated accordingly.
- Neurological deficits or progression of deficits is indications for surgery. If the patient has neurological deficits or progressing neurological impairment, I strongly recommend considering surgery to avoid nerve damage that could be permanent.

When recommending a specific conservative or surgical treatment, the decision for surgery may rely on medical data. EBM should be applied. A spine surgeon may recommend a treatment other than the "conventional management" outlined in guidelines and algorithms.

Myths in the Treatment of Patients with LBP

These are the most frequent myths:

- Back surgery will cause further deterioration of the spine. (This is not necessarily true, but fusion surgery may accelerate deterioration of the spine.)
- Life will be different after back surgery. I tell my patients it is not because they had surgery what changes their life. It is because an injury caused spinal damage and life will never be the same, but it is not that surgery has a negative effect on people's lives. Surgery increased the chances for improvement and for getting back into a reasonably active life.
- People say that, "if there is not a hundred percent chance of improvement after surgery, I had better stay the same". This statement is wrong. There are patients who had back surgery and have no more symptoms. (This is mostly if patients are compliant with the surgeon's recommendations.) If a surgeon does not guarantee one hundred percent chance for improvement, I am not having back surgery. This is also wrong.

There is virtually no surgeon who can guarantee one hundred percent improvement even if we, as surgeons, have cases with one hundred percent improvement. The problem I see with this attitude is that there is a greater chance for complications for not having surgery. Delayed surgery is also related to some complications related to scar tissue formation and worsening of a spinal conditions, making surgery more difficult than if done earlier.

- Surgery at a large center guarantees better surgical outcome. This is not true. A local surgeon should be qualified to perform spine surgery. If the local surgeon does not feel comfortable with certain procedures, the same surgeon will refer you to a "large center." Ironically, patients sometimes receive more personal and quality treatment at their hometown than at "large centers."

- Some people dislike doctors and hospitals. This is a negative generalization. Mistakes and other adverse outcomes occur in hospitals, but one cannot generalize these situations. One, as a patient, should check certain aspects of the hospital, nurses, and doctors in the community. It is wrong to suffer pain only because of misconceptions.

- Old age is a contraindication for surgery. Wrong! This is also a misconception. However, one must check with the surgeon for a preoperative medical evaluation.

- There is no remedy for a spinal condition. Patients say, "I already underwent two surgeries (or more), and I am still in pain." It is true the more operations, the less favorable the prognosis. However, I would not say a patient is doomed to be in pain for life. I remember a man who had had eight back surgeries prior to our consultation. I found the cause of pain and did his surgery. The patient got significantly better to the point that he did not require any pain medication. There is also the alternative of a "pain clinic" in which certain procedures may alleviate pain.

- Patients tell me, "I have diabetes. I am too old and in bad shape for surgery. I do not think that I will make it through surgery alive." Once again, as a surgeon, one can do a preoperative evaluation or send a patient to a cardiologist or an internist for a medical evaluation before surgery. Surgery can still be undertaken in some cases, or there can be other surgical alternatives.

- A patient should have two months or more of conservative treatment before considering surgery. I have extensively talked about indications for surgery. Review this section of the book. There is not necessarily a specific time for surgery. Each patient is different and should be treated accordingly.

- Because a patient has severe pain, emergency surgery is warranted. Wrong! The fact that a patient is in severe pain does not necessarily mean the patient should have emergency surgery. I have seen patients in my office with severe back and leg pain showing signs of nerve irritation (leg pain), but the radiological studies are negative and fail to show nerve impingement. Many of these patients may have a great deal of pain from muscle spasm because of a strain/sprain. Surgeons must be cautious when recommending surgery. There are other causes of severe back pain, such as sacral-iliac joint dysfunction and facet joint syndrome. These can be very painful and can simulate a ruptured disc and sciatica. Patients should also be cautious of surgeons who are quick to do surgery and have a reputation for "performing rushed surgeries."

- One would distrust a surgeon only because he or she is not American Board Certified. Be cautious when judging a physician for his or her aspect, ethnic background, or board certification status. American board certification does not guarantee better care.

- Physical therapy is needed after surgery. Physical therapy is not always necessary before or after surgery. Each patient is different. I have had patients who did not require any kind of "rehabilitation" because of the good outcome.

- Epidural shots before surgery are always indicated. Wrong! I have already elaborated about epidural blocks in the treatment chapter. Actually, epidural blocks may increase the chances for intraoperative complications because of scar tissue formation and the increased risk of spinal fluid leak from dura tears. I have already mentioned that epidural blocks for LBP patients are still controversial and are falling out of favor.

Other Medical Issues

New advancements place a special twist in the practice of medicine and particularly in the case of surgery. How does a surgeon get updated on current surgical techniques after a surgical residency? I have already answered these questions in my previous discussion of indications for surgery.

There are special courses and seminars that physicians attend. However, the questions are: Does a "weekend course" enable a surgeon to start practicing a new surgical technique? Does a surgeon have to have a full year of training to "learn" the new technique? Do patients always have to go to university hospitals or those with a certain reputation and where research is carried out all the time? Is a patient safe in a university hospital where, not only new surgical techniques are developed, but also there are novice surgeons? These questions are difficult to answer. Only a surgeon who is honest with his or her work and capabilities can address and decide these issues.

The downside of newer surgical techniques is there can be complications that are by far more difficult than the disease itself. The patient has to make a decision for surgery with strong, careful considerations and with a clear mind. If a surgeon has learned spine surgery during his or her training or residency and the surgeon has a high surgical success rate on his or her patients, the same surgeon can learn new techniques and apply them appropriately. The surgeon has to be honest about his or her limitations.

As long as the surgeon feels confident with the personnel, the equipment, his or her skills, and the new surgical technique, the odds for complications should be the same as the any other surgical technique. However, it may be recommended having a surgeon who has done more complex surgeries operate with the surgeon who is learning a new technique.

However, one must be cautious because there are certain surgical techniques that are more complex with a high degree of risk. They require more sophisticated equipment, personnel training, and other specialists involved in a particular case. The surgeon must be honest enough to admit a particular case is more complicated and cannot be handled at a particular institution.

Science attempts to challenge the laws of mechanics and to defy our relentless biological clocks. But, that is all they are—attempts. There is no perfect solution for the complicated paradigm in the treatment of a patient with LBP. It is unfortunate that science can sometimes cause more harm while attempting to solve complicated problems. Studies are performed prior to implementing treatments for patients with LBP and other medical conditions. The problems we face with these studies can generally be attributed to alterations, inaccuracies related to bias, and other factors not taken into consideration when performing the studies. One must be cautious when interpreting the information provided by a particular scientific article or publication.

Questions

What alternatives do I have for the treatment of my lower back pain? There are essentially five options:

1. No treatment at all
2. Conservative treatment

3. Semiconservative invasive treatment

4. Surgery

5. Gene therapy (stem-cell)

We can fairly separate LBP treatment into three main categories: conservative, semiconservative, and surgical. Semiconservative treatment is rapidly evolving. There have been relatively new advances in the treatment of spine conditions in which the patient is treated more aggressively than with simple conservative measures, but it does not involve surgery.

By semiconservative treatment, I mean new treatment techniques that involve needles, probes, catheters, and so forth. These techniques can be invasive, and they can be subject to complications. Patient must sign a surgical consent for surgery and semiconservative procedures.

I do not recommend neglecting treatment for someone with LBP. I think that, if our body is experiencing pain, it is telling us that something is imbalanced (trauma, strain/sprain, and so forth), and there is a need for treatment. However, if the pain is only minimal or mild, if it is subsiding (in one or two days), and it is not affecting a young person, there will probably be no need for a medical visit. An aspirin or anti-inflammatory medication and little bed rest will relieve the pain.

Conservative treatment does not involve any invasive procedures such as spinal injections or surgery. Physical therapy, water exercises, hypnosis, complementary and alternative medicine, low back exercises, and even pain medications and muscle relaxants can be considered as "conservative treatment."

Semiconservative treatment is conservative treatment combined with spinal injections ("spinal shot" or epidural block, trigger point injections, facet joint blocks, nerve block, IDET, spinal stimulator implants, morphine pump implant, adhenolysis, and so forth). These treatments carry an increased risk of complications when compared with conservative treatment (related to the use of invasive procedures).

There is always the risk of complications related to surgery. Certain surgical procedures carry a higher risk than others do. A surgeon should explain the variants and alternatives for different surgical procedures, their complications, and the experience of the surgeon on each technique.

Gene therapy is still in an experimental phase.

Is it possible that the disc will heal without any treatment at all? Yes. However, a patient should not procrastinate and neglect the treatment of a lower back condition. I recommend professional (medical) treatment and advice.

It is my observation that some patients who develop a disc herniation heal. The disc spontaneously shrinks and even disappears (absorbs) with time (unspecified) in some occasions. However, there is no way to predict when the herniated disc will heal spontaneously. It may take six months or more. During this time, a compressed nerve can be permanently damaged. I would not recommend waiting for the disc "to heal by itself." I would recommend consulting a spine specialist.

There are new studies related to the natural history of a disc herniation on a patient. The results are yet not conclusive. It is my observation that young patients in their twenties tend to have spontaneous disc rupture absorption, but in the case of disc herniation on patients older than thirty, the ruptured disc tends to either stay the same, get larger, or even calcify. Patients older than sixty do not tend to absorb a ruptured disc spontaneously. The phenomena may be related to the capacity of the body to heal easier and faster when young. The tissues may still have a significant amount of water and collagen tissue as well as macrophages and other defensive reactions of the body to injury in the young patient. Spontaneous disc absorption can occur in as little as six or eight weeks. However, the pain in the lower back and the legs may persist after spontaneous disc absorption. The kind of disc that tends to absorb spontaneously is the "free fragment disc," but not the contained herniated disc.

Currently, there is no clear predictive data to support certain treatments for patients with LBP. A patient with a large disc herniation will likely have a great deal of pain (low back and/or leg pain) and neurological deficits. This patient should be treated. A patient with a large disc herniation who has no surgery may develop more symptoms, or the disc may break. Then the "free fragment" may cause more symptoms or may be absorbed spontaneously with no particular treatment. These patients may be at risk for nerve damage if treatment is delayed. There is no clear data to predict which group of patients will get worse in time and which ones will improve and "heal" spontaneously. Recent studies address this issue; however, no clear data predicts which patients with "small disc herniation" will end up in surgery. Several factors influence the predictive information.

Do I need back surgery? A spine surgeon will explain any issues related to surgery, including indications, success rate, complications, rehabilitation, recovery time, physical limitations and activities after surgery, medication side effects, wound care, special use of braces, and so forth. The decision for treatment, especially for surgery, should be made relying on what is called EBM. EBM is the analysis summary of all factors involved with a particular patient, plus the medical data and common sense. There is no "best" surgery for patients with the same condition. Certain surgical techniques may apply best for certain people. One of the most common mistakes I have seen in my practice is that a surgeon treats a condition (MRI, X-rays, and so forth)—not a patient.

If I need surgery, what kind of surgery do I need? One must consider several factors when choosing a specific surgical technique. Probably the most common influence on the surgeon to choose one surgery over another is the reliance on scientific information (textbooks, articles, and medical journals dedicated to the spine). Some of this information has flaws. Studies review only certain aspects of the patient with LBP, but there are no randomized prospective studies on patients with one specific spinal disorder with exactly the same biological, clinical presentation, radiological studies, and social and cultural characteristics. One must consider the following when trying to decide about surgery:

- Studies usually group patients with LBP under one category. We have seen that there are many causes of LBP; therefore, the treatment varies.

- Patients with LBP from a herniated disc may not be treated the same way. Some patients with LBP, leg pain, and a herniated disc may need surgery very soon, and others may not need surgery at all. Here is where the art and experience of the surgeon becomes of paramount importance.

- Companies that manufacture medical instruments are always pressing to sell their products based also on questionable studies, and they may influence surgeons in the decision-making process.

- Bear in mind that surgeons charge according to the procedure.

- It is up to the surgeon to decide the type of surgery to be performed, but the patient should understand first the indications for the surgery. The goal is then to be achieved with the recommended surgery. However, the patient should be given the most common options for treatment, indications, and complications as well as the reasons for recommending certain treatment.

These issues are important because the decision for surgery and the type of procedure should be tailored for that particular patient. Patients have different personalities, psychology, lifestyle, work, and expectations. A surgeon must consider all variants and see the patient as a whole to decide which procedure is more suitable for the patient.

The problem with performing the surgery that was not exactly the best choice for a patient is that it may carry complications or an adverse outcome. A patient may experience more LBP after back surgery. There can be serious complications with aggressive surgeries. "Failed back surgery syndrome" may lead to subsequent operations.

If I have back surgery, will I need another operation in the future? Patients ask me this question frequently. They say, "I will never be the same." Does another surgery always guarantee improvement, or will there be further deterioration of the spine?

To answer these questions, we must consider several factors, such as age, smoking history, obesity, body habits and posture, type of back condition, underlying factors (for example, the naturally deterioration of the spine), type of surgical technique used during the first or subsequent surgeries, and so forth.

What questions should I ask my family physician and my surgeon? There are questions that are pertinent and appropriate to ask the primary care physician and surgeon.

These questions would be appropriate to ask the primary care physician: Has the primary care physician known the surgeon several years? Is the surgeon reliable? One must remember that personal conflicts between primary care physicians and surgeons sometimes interfere with quality care for the patient. When the surgeon is competent and honest, but the primary care physician refers the patient to another surgeon, whether local or out of town, the patient suffers the inconvenience and consequences only because of personal matters between physicians. Therefore, one must be cautious when following the primary care physician's advice. We have to remember that physicians may have biased opinions due to personal problems or other reasons (prejudice). The primary care physician may not send his or her patients to a particular surgeon, even if the surgeon is competent and is located geographically within a convenient distance for the patient.

Another situation I have encountered is when a patient says his or her primary care physician recommended surgery but the surgeon disagreed. There are primary care physicians who like to give "surgical advice," but they have neither the experience nor the training of a surgeon. However, the primary care physician may infer, anticipate, or suspect there is the possibility of surgery. That is why they send the patient to the surgeon for a surgical consultation.

I have seen patients who tell me: "You are my second opinion." "My doctor (primary care physician) told me I need surgery. You said the same so that makes you my second opinion." Insurance companies and surgeons understand "second opinion" as another surgeon's opinion.

Patients sometimes get frustrated because I recommend more studies or a referral to another specialist. They feel they have "wasted their time" coming to me. It is important the primary care physician explain to the patient the reason for a referral to a spine surgeon and to tell the patient what to expect from the consultation.

Other questions to ask the surgeon can be related to medical background. Some people think medical schools train surgeons to practice. They do not realize that medical school is important, but what gives a physician the training is a specific program for the preparation and education related to a medical specialty (residency training program).

It is ironic that foreign medical graduate physicians are distrusted because of their medical background. Many foreign physicians have already completed residency training in their countries. By the time the physician gets into an American residency training program, that physician has a great deal of experience and has done the same residency twice. A physician that is not American Board Certified can be as qualified and competent as one that is.

One must be cautious with another misleading situation. Some people think that, because a physician is a graduate of a reputable medical school and/or training program, he or she is/or should be a top-quality surgeon. There is no doubt the large reputable universities and hospitals have high academic standards. But it is also true that, at some programs, physicians-in-training do not have ample exposure to the practice of surgery because of the legal system. Experience and skill is gained over years of practice.

One must trust the basic medical background information, but one should also consider the principles of EBM as well as the physician's experience and honesty.

A patient may ask a surgeon about surgical outcome and success rate. Other questions can be related to the reasons for the decision of a particular recommended surgery. Expectancies, recovery time, work status, physical limitations, and so forth are also valid issues to address.

The treating physician should know which surgical or medical codes to use for billing and collection purposes. Physicians and patients must be familiar with ICD-9 and CPT codes.

If a physician (including the surgeon) is offended by the questions, the patient can always find another surgeon who will answer reasonable questions related to the surgery, options, hospital stay, rehabilitation, and physical limitations. The surgeon should not become defensive or get offended. The patient is entitled to ask about the surgeon's background and experience, success rate, complications, and so forth. If the surgeon feels uncomfortable with the "questioning of his abilities or credentials," he or she should manage the situation in the following way, "I have enough training and experience in knowing how to perform your surgery, and I am prepared to deal with any complication."

Do not be afraid to ask questions related to work status, physical activities, expected pain, wound care, sex, medical expenses, surgical assistant, and even the type of anesthesia to be used. The patient can also obtain information about the anesthesiologist (medical background, experience, and so forth). The patient should direct these questions to the anesthesiologist. Typically, the anesthesiologist will contact the patient before surgery to ask some medical questions. Ask the anesthesiologist about adverse effects or side effects to anesthesia.

Ask questions regarding financial arrangements to the physician's office staff. There is nothing more unpleasant than to have a happy patient with a satisfactory postoperative outcome and a negative attitude because of extra charges not considered prior to the surgery.

When asking for medical background and credentials, one must be reasonable and not suspicious of the surgeon. Explain that you feel entitled to know some information on the surgeon and physicians involved in surgery. If the patient knows the surgeon on a personal basis or simply by "word of mouth," the patient may feel very confident of the surgeon and may avoid all of these questions that may create some conflict with the surgeon.

I have wondered why we, as physicians, have to comply with very strict norms because we treat people and their lives are in our hands. But there are certain professions in which we also put our lives at risk, and nobody questions any educational background, skill, training, experience, qualifications, and so forth. We take for granted they know what they are doing. Pilots, attorneys, bus drivers, architects, and so forth, we trust them with our lives. Yet, very rarely, do we ever ask them for their "credentials." This is one of those ironies of life.

What about recovery? Ask the surgeon these questions because recovery may vary, depending on the type of surgery performed. Some studies encourage "outpatient" surgery nowadays. I still have not reached that point because I still believe back surgery is a major procedure from which dangerous complications may arise in the first twenty-four to forty-eight hours. Therefore, I typically keep my patients in the hospital for at least twenty-four hours, but I decide how long a patient stays, depending on their response, not only physical but also psychological. I have discharged patients from the hospital on the same day of surgery. It all depends on the patient's attitude, response to surgery, pain control, and so forth.

Less hospital stay will lower the chances for infections and other complications. Twenty-four to forty-eight hours is a reasonable time for a patient to stay after back surgery, regardless of the age. However, hospital stay depends also on the type of surgery, complications, and other issues. The elderly can be transferred to another ward for early rehabilitation, such as rehabilitation centers, step-down units, transitional care units, and even nursing homes.

There is open surgery, and there is endoscopic surgery. In my opinion, both may require the patient to stay at least overnight to monitor for complications and treat them promptly. This management is the surgeon's preference.

I strongly believe patients recover faster in their own home environment. Not to mention that, in the hospital, patients can be exposed to infections, noise, and lack of sleep that could lower the immune system. After all, surgery is an aggression to the body from which it has to recover with appropriate sleep, food, and quiet environment. I give about two to three weeks for the wound to heal. After that, I may place the patient in a program of physical therapy. However, the day after surgery, I encourage them to do range-of-motion exercises for the legs and hips in bed. I believe that early, light exercising promotes healing and boosts the immune system.

Do doctors know everything about LBP? The answer is no! Not all about every disease is known. In fact, there are always evolving changes in medicine every day. Furthermore, not all physicians know everything about low back problems. However, general practitioners should be aware of the newest trends in treatments.

How are physicians updated in the newest or latest medical advances? Physicians must comply with certain regulations to be able to practice medicine. One of the main regulations is to have a current medical license. In order to keep a medical license updated and current, there is a need for "credits" or continuing medical education (CME). Physicians must take special courses and seminars in their specialty to accumulate certain number of CME hours to renew a medical license and maintain hospital privileges. Most physicians are also subscribed to prestigious medical journals, publications, and reviews.

How do I choose my surgeon? Medical boards, state boards, and other associations have a way of "disciplining" physicians who have incurred too many adverse outcomes on patients. Hospitals have a special committee assigned for "quality assurance." Sometimes, it is called "performance improvement." These committees are designed to "police" physicians and to inquire the reasons for adverse outcomes. Members of the committee are in charge of following patterns. If there is a pattern of complications and adverse outcomes with a physician, the committee is in charge of confronting and dealing with any situation. Specialty medical boards usually do not "police" physicians. One must be careful when judging a physician because of "too many" adverse outcomes. Adverse outcomes can be expected in certain difficult patients.

Physicians who deal with complex cases might expect a "high" adverse outcome rate. Patients that are a high risk for infection and other complications are considered when "looking" into a physician's complication rate. Board certification by a medical specialty does not ensure a physician is competent. More board-certified physicians can have a high complication rate than non-board certified physicians. Word of mouth is probably one of the best ways of finding a competent physician. Once again, one must be cautious when judging and selecting a physician. Primary care physicians might not refer a patient to a particular specialist due to personal conflicts or other personal issues. One must not base judgment on what one patient says about a physician. One patient might have had a bad experience with the office or the hospital. Or simply, the patient might be demanding and abusive and might give a bad reference about a physician. Several comments are better than only one or two isolated comments about a physician.

What is the recovery time, hospital stay, work status, and so forth? Will I need to wear a brace after surgery? Recovery time after back surgery is variable. It is relative to the type of surgery that has been performed. What I recommend to my patients who underwent low back surgery without fusion (microdiskectomy or microdiscectomy) is that it takes three weeks to heal and to increase physical activity progressively. After three weeks of light physical activities, I may let the patient start driving within a radius of about ten miles. Sitting, standing, and walking for more than thirty minutes should be avoided because the patient may experience LBP from muscle spasm and rigidity.

The soft tissues, ligaments, and muscles will still be swollen and tender from surgery for the first three to six weeks (or more). I may send a patient to physical therapy three weeks after the surgery. I usually recommend physical therapy three times per week for four to six or even eight weeks.

If the patient had a spinal bone fusion with no instrumentation, I recommend wearing a hard (plastic) back brace for about three months. For patients who had spinal instrumentation (hardware with screws, plates, or rods), there are different preferences. Some surgeons do not prescribe a back brace; others do. Traveling during the first eight weeks is not recommended. Surgeons at certain institutions do disc surgery as an outpatient procedure, and the patient goes home on the same day of surgery.

Work status during the recovery time is an issue I address after the first postoperative visit. Work status is also related to the kind of work the patient does, the physical constitution, and other variants. I will further discuss work status in the workers' compensation section.

How can I avoid worsening my low back condition? Will my back continue to deteriorate? Use common sense to avoid low back injuries. Avoid factors and activities that could aggravate the lower back condition or reinjure yourself. Take responsibility and control over contributing factors to the development of LBP, such as obesity, smoking, and strenuous activities. Stay in good physical condition.

As part of the normal natural aging process, the spine continues to deteriorate. We have to consider some of these aspects when answering questions regarding the future treatment of the patient with a low back injury. Certain surgical procedures (spinal fusion with instrumentation) have been proven to accelerate the deterioration rate at other levels in the spine by increasing physical stress on the adjacent joints. These are some suggestions I have for my patients to slow the deterioration process of the spine:

- Avoid activities that could cause further wearing of the spine, such as bending, twisting, or lifting (heavy objects or objects heavier than thirty-five pounds). (Please refer to the chapter on ergonomics and mechanics of the spine.)

- Follow a regular program of exercise and diet.

- Avoid smoking, certain foods, obesity, and activities that could cause early deterioration of the bones and joints. (Obesity has not been proven to increase spinal deterioration; however, I do recommend avoiding obesity in general.)

- Treat underlying joint or bone conditions, such as osteoporosis, rheumatoid arthritis, diabetes, obesity, and so forth.

Why do some patients benefit from low back surgery and others do not? Will I be one who benefits or one who fails or gets worse from surgery? Again, the outcome of surgery varies. It depends on the type of injury, disease, or disorder. The outcome depends on the kind of surgery utilized and other factors plus underlying conditions, such as smoking, diabetes, obesity, osteoporosis, and so forth.

This is a complex question in which all factors involved with an individual are taken into consideration, such as age, work, physical constitution, habits, primary spinal problem, and timing of treatment.

The results may be very good following surgery. As time goes by, the success rate tends to decline. I have noticed that, in time (one to two years), some patients develop recurrent LBP and even leg pain. This phenomenon can be related to a number of factors:

- Lack of compliance (negligence)
- Scar tissue formation
- Obesity, smoking, and poor mechanical factors
- Lack of exercises on a regular basis
- Natural further deterioration of the spine (aging)
- Re-injury

These are some of the most common reasons for someone to develop recurrent pain. Scar tissue formation may be the most frequent cause of recurrent pain. Surgery is not accepted as a treatment for scar tissue formation. Most recently, studies have been made in the use of radiotherapy for scar tissue formation with positive results. More prospective studies will be needed to establish safety and positive results.

Many patients with recurrent symptoms will need another MRI scan, but few will have a real problem that will require surgery. However, more aggressive surgeons will recommend a spinal fusion for the "further deteriorated spine," patients with scar tissue formation, or patients with degenerative disc disease (DDD). Some of the common rules for treatment and statistical data are controversial because studies include all patients with LBP without separating population variables.

In order to obtain more consistent and accurate data, there would have to be several studies in which certain groups of patients are followed for several years. Otherwise, information on low back conditions may be misleading if the studies are not properly randomized and selected by individual groups (for example, age, location of the lesion, general conditions, type of work, and litigation issues). There are reliable studies in some of the well-known journals of spine in which, most recently, these issues have been addressed and analyzed, making the data more accurate. Primary care physicians rely significantly on medical journals and experts' opinion. These opinions are often based on studies rather than on the personal experience of a spine surgeon. In my opinion, this experience is of utmost significance when treating patients with spine conditions. Clinical studies and journals are excellent sources of basic medical information, but we cannot rely one hundred percent on these studies. Not only because they may be biased or confusing, but external sources may have be altered or manipulated the data.

Treating a patient with a spinal condition is a complex field because the current literature dictates early rehabilitation, conservative treatment, and surgery as the last resort. What is an appropriate time for conservative treatment before considering surgery? Again, it all depends on the cause of pain and other medical conditions. Four to six weeks of conservative treatment before considering surgery cannot always be applied to the patient with LBP. This approach should not always be a standard rule for the treatment of a patient with LBP.

How long will my surgeon see me after surgery? There is no rule on the time a surgeon will see a patient after surgery. Each surgeon has a routine for the follow-up of patients after surgery. There are surgeons who let the PA, NP, or medical assistant see the patient in the postoperative stage. Only if there is a concern, the surgeon will see the patient. There are times when the surgeon sees the patient a couple of times after surgery. Then a medical assistant will follow the patient.

Typically, insurance companies reimburse the surgeon for the operation and for what they consider a "global period after surgery," which is typically three months. There are times when insurance companies do not even pay the surgeon for work done before surgery because it is included in the "global period."

Surgeons typically follow the patient for about three months. Then, if no more surgery is needed, the patient is discharged from the surgeon's care to follow with the primary care physician (referring). If the patient did not have a primary care physician, the surgeon can assist the patient in getting a primary care physician. In the case of workers' compensation patients, a primary doctor (occupational or industrial medicine specialist) will usually follow the patient, sometimes for a few weeks after surgery. However, every surgeon has preferences. I follow patients for as long as I must. I have sometimes followed patients for as long as six months or more. The need for extended follow-up also depends on the system and the particular setting in town.

Some insurance companies (workers' compensation) want the surgeon follow patients for several months because they consider the surgeon as the primary care physician. Thus, the surgeon orders physical therapy, assistance devices, medications, and so forth until the surgeon discharges the patient. Some primary care physicians feel uncomfortable treating a patient who sustained a work-related injury. Some primary care physicians are also unfamiliar with forms and terms used in the workers' compensation system and have the surgeon do all the paperwork. Eventually, the surgeon will discharge the patient. If the patient still has symptoms, the surgeon may refer the patient to a pain clinic for pain management. Or, if the patient was already addicted to pain medications before surgery, the patient may require rehabilitation.

Typically, surgeons prescribe certain medications after surgery for a few weeks, but the primary care physician, a pain specialist, or the occupational medicine practitioner will follow the patient for nonsurgical treatment. The surgeon usually sends reports of the follow-up visits to the referring or primary care physician to keep him or her informed of the patient's progress, plans, and treatment. I usually send copies of my follow-up reports (and the first consultation) to the primary care physician and the insurance company (in the case of workers' compensation).

A frequent situation I have experienced is when a patient has back surgery. The patient improves from the symptoms. Several months or years later, the patient experiences back pain again. The primary care physician refers the patient back to the surgeon without even examining the patient, without any studies, and without any treatment, regardless of the symptoms' severity. Only because the patient had back surgery, the spine surgeon should see the patient again. It is my experience that, in the majority of the cases, the patient does not require further surgery, but only primary care.

CHAPTER 6

Rehabilitation

Rehabilitation (Before and After Back Surgery)

Rehabilitation is a very important part of the treatment of LBP patients and starts even before surgery. There is also rehabilitation for the nonsurgical patient who had a low back injury. Patients benefit from rehabilitation if started soon after the injury. Patients tend to believe surgery is the total solution rather than viewing it as part of the treatment.

There are important aspects of rehabilitation that play a role in the outcome of a patient with LBP:

- Patient's compliance, body constitution and frame, habits, and underlying medical conditions
- **The surgeon.** Selected surgery, professionalism, experience, knowledge, and competency.
- **Rehabilitation.** Physical therapists and their competency.

If these elements are not applied to the patient with LBP, there is a good chance for a poor outcome. The success of surgery does not rest only on one of the above factors.

Rehabilitation is so important that no rehabilitation at all or the wrong type of rehabilitation can hinder the other significant elements during the course of treatment. The same applies to the other elements of the equation. If one of the elements fails, chances are there will be poor results.

Rehabilitation is a period of time before or after surgery or after an injury (in which surgery was not required), in which certain types of treatment are carried out, such as physical therapy, occupational therapy, improved body mechanics, biofeedback (when indicated), detoxification, as well as motivation and psychological counseling. During rehabilitation, a patient may use mild painkillers and other pharmacological treatments. Types of rehabilitation would include retraining, occupational therapy, "work hardening," vocational rehabilitation, and so forth. When we speak of rehabilitation, we refer not only to physical therapy after surgery, but to other aspects of treatment.

It is also important to emphasize there are different types and applications of physical therapy. This is one of the most common mistakes physicians make when treating a patient with LBP. Physicians send their patient for physical therapy with the diagnosis of "low back pain," but they do not specify the kind of therapy ordered for a specific patient (with a specific back condition).

Physical therapy has to be tailored to a specific patient. When recommending rehabilitation, we must consider other aspects such as economic status and social situation. Some patients cannot drive and have no assistance; some cannot travel for other reasons. Sometimes, patients do not believe in physical therapy and rehabilitation. They think they will be hurt more. Unfortunately, this is true. Patients are sometimes injured through certain phases of rehabilitation and physical therapy.

Physical therapists also have the idea that all patients with LBP should be treated the same way. They apply the same exercises and treatment to all patients. (Please refer to the chapter in conservative treatment and modified low back exercises.)

The following are some of my recommendations for physical activities, positions, posture, and exercises for the person with LBP and for the patient who had any kind of low back surgery. These exercises are to be performed only under the supervision of a physician and at the appropriate time after surgery.

Low Back Exercises

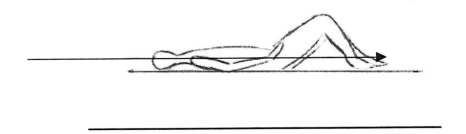

When exercising, one must remember to keep the spine aligned and straight—no matter what kind of exercises the person is performing. It is also better to keep the spine (back) supported against a flat surface.

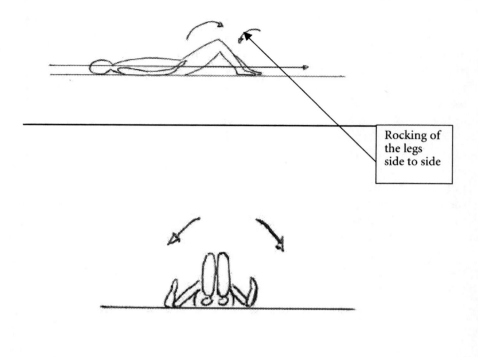

Rocking of
the legs
side to side

This is an exercise in which the knees are bent and there is slight, comfortable rocking of the legs from side to side. This is an excellent exercise to relieve sacroiliac joint pain. This exercise can be performed in repetitions of five, ten, or twenty. I do twenty repetitions. I then switch to other type of exercises and before coming back and doing the same exercise twenty times again.

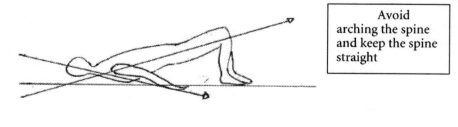

Avoid
arching the spine
and keep the spine
straight

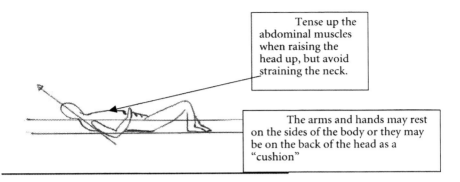

Tense up the abdominal muscles when raising the head up, but avoid straining the neck.

The arms and hands may rest on the sides of the body or they may be on the back of the head as a "cushion"

This is an excellent exercise to strengthen the abdominal muscles, and it is a variant of the abdominal crunches. I do not recommend classical abdominal crunches for people with LBP who had surgery. One must be careful not to bend the neck in order to avoid any strain on it. Keep the neck aligned with the head as shown with the arrows. This particular exercise is also very helpful for the pelvis muscles. No matter what exercise one performs, avoid overarching the lumbar spine either way.

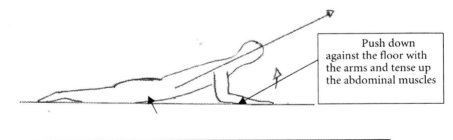

Push down against the floor with the arms and tense up the abdominal muscles

One must be careful with this exercise in order to avoid overextension of the spine (neck and back). A modification to this exercise is a slight raising of the head off the floor and tensing up the abdominal muscles.

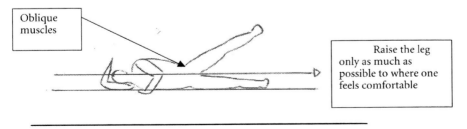

Oblique muscles

Raise the leg only as much as possible to where one feels comfortable

This exercise is excellent to strengthen the oblique muscles. When working out and trying to strengthen the muscles to support the spine, one must work in all muscles around the spine: the front (abdominal muscles), the back, and the sides (oblique muscles). This is also a good exercise to strengthen the hip muscles. Avoid tilting the head up or down in order to avoid any straining when performing this exercise.

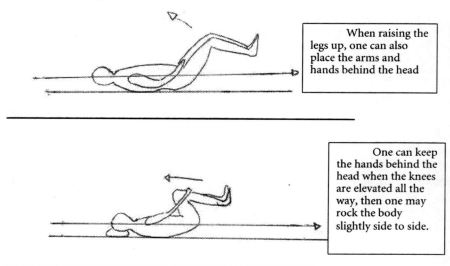

When raising the legs up, one can also place the arms and hands behind the head

One can keep the hands behind the head when the knees are elevated all the way, then one may rock the body slightly side to side.

This is an exercise to strengthen the abdominal muscles and the psoas muscle.

Body Mechanics. When performing any activity, no matter what, one must keep the spine straight and aligned with the head and the pelvis. These are only a few activities to demonstrate the axis of the body and how the body must be always kept:

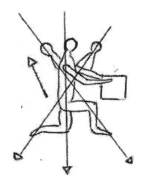

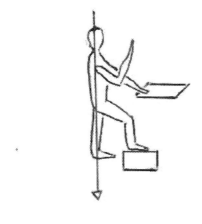

It is always a good idea to use a step stool to prop one leg up when standing. This helps the lower back take some of the strain off the spine.

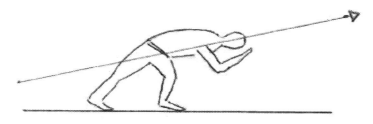

When leaning forward, by keeping one leg outstretched and the other bent at the knee, one takes strain off the lower back.

The above exercises and postures are only examples. Books, magazines, and other literature provide extensive guides for proper body mechanics and for low back exercises. However, one must be cautious with the exercises recommended by some physical therapist, back specialist, and other health care providers. Some exercises may cause more LBP. I will address more modifications to low back exercises, body mechanics, posture, sports, and gym activities in another edition (and/or DVD) in the future.

There are exercises that traditionally have been recommended for patients with LBP for several years, such as the "McKenzie" exercises and other routine therapy. These traditional "back exercises" are not indicated to all patients with

LBP. There are different causes of LBP among patients. Physical therapy must have not only scientific support, but common sense is primordial.

Preventing Back Injuries

One of the best approaches to the patient with LBP is to prevent the development of LBP in the first place. All human beings have common sense, but we sometimes neglect it.

By following medical advice and considering some facts, we may be able to prevent serious injuries. These are some preventive observations and measurements to avoid low back injuries:

- Many accidents happen during the first hours of the day. Be especially cautions and careful during this time of the day.

- Avoid doing activities to "cut corners" that neglect doing activities the safe way.

- Avoid pure negligence.

- Educate people in general about the mechanics of the spine. Ignorance and lack of body mechanics is one of the main reasons that accidents happen.

- Avoid poor judgment and lack of consideration for possible risks.

- Fatigue and exhaustion may lead to sloppiness and make people prone to accidents. Avoid getting into the situation of extreme exhaustion.

- Improve safety guidelines.

- Maintain good physical fitness and avoid bad habits such as smoking and excessive eating (obesity) or other noxious activities and habits.

Physicians, nurses, safety managers, and engineers work constantly to improve working conditions to decrease the chances for work-related accidents or occupational-related disorders. Some companies have posters and other information posted for employees to read and follow. Employees should have more frequent sessions or classes of safety conditions, prevention, and body ergonomics to avoid work injuries.

Employees should be rotated periodically to avoid repetitive work that can cause strain to body parts. General fitness should be encouraged to employees, possibly with the construction of gyms and other areas of fitness. Offer diet classes led by dieticians and other activities to maintain general good health. A program of regular back exercises for employees with back injuries should be implemented. Counselors, psychologists, and psychiatrists should be involved whenever there is aggression in the workplace. Job dissatisfaction should be worked out. Job dissatisfaction is one of the most frequent problems associated with patients suffering with LBP. Prevention is the key in medicine.

More Comments Related to LBP Treatment

Some physicians think an internal disruption of the disc can cause "discogenic pain." It has been proven that there are indeed micro tears due to microtrauma to the disc that have been seen microscopically. Pain specialists, in an attempt to describe in layman's terms a disc herniation, explain this disruption as a "leaking disc." This term often confuses patients I see in my office. They want to know if the disc is still "leaking." They want me to explain to them what the other physician meant by a "leaking disc." To my surprise, patients do not ask the same questions to their treating physicians or they receive a too simple explanation or an explanation with medical technical terms they do not clearly understand. Patients sometimes get a technically complex explanation of a disc herniation. Patients deserve an explanation in layman's terms.

Scientific data shows that, when there is an annular tear in the disc, there is also chemical irritation of the nerve by the content of the disc itself. Sometimes, there is only degenerative disc disease and a mild bulging disc. In these cases, there is no clear cause of the symptoms of leg pain.

There is controversy on the source of LBP and leg pain. Many other factors contribute to the cause of LBP and leg pain, such as psychological factors, secondary gain, obesity, and so forth. Some surgeons believe that, because there is an "internal derangement" of the disc, there is a need for a spinal fusion. They call this condition discogenic disease, and fusion surgery is done. We refer to this condition as DDD or degenerative disc disease.

I have seen many patients with low back and leg pain, but their MRI scans show only mild DDD or a bulging disc. Some of these patients are obese, smoke, have poor posture and bad habits, do not use body mechanics, and have LBP. When a report of a lumbar spine reads terms such as bulging disc, degenerative disc disease, and so forth, the situation gets confusing for everybody—the patient, physician, surgeon, and insurance companies. Some patients have only what is read by a radiologist on an MRI report, "mild spinal stenosis or small bulging disc." The MRI scan might show as much as forty-six to ninety percent "DDD" on patients ages fifty to sixty. On patients over sixty years of age, the chances of detecting DDD by MRI scan are close to ninety percent.

On the other hand, when obese patients have a lumbar spine MRI scan, they lay down flat on the MRI machine table. We do not know the dynamics of the spine if the patient was standing. If a patient is in the reclining position, the MRI scan shows a bulging disc. In real time, an MRI scan on the same person while standing will show the true size of the disc protrusion, and we will be able to see how much the disc is pressing the nerves. The disc that seems to be mildly bulging on a MRI scan would probably bulge out more in the standing position if we could get an MRI scan in the standing position. This is probably the reason that physicians sometimes "cannot explain" the patient's severe pain if the MRI scan shows "only a small bulging disc."

There are new machines and studies under investigation for dynamic MRI scans. New MRI machines are starting to be developed that show the spine in real time and shape. To my knowledge, there are not valid studies that predict the future of the spine when an MRI scan shows degenerative changes. No one knows with certainty that patients with abnormal MRI scans will need back surgery in the future. However, there have been times in which I have followed patients for years, and, with the association of the patient's symptoms, radiological studies (MRI scans), and the progression of the disease over time, I can predict some changes of the spine in the future on certain patients.

I think it is unfair that some surgeons do not do surgery on a patient with LBP, leg pain, spinal stenosis, and/or a disc herniation because the patient is obese. It is true it is recommended the patient lose weight, but the reality is that many patients are obese precisely because they cannot engage in a program of sports or strenuous physical activities. Many of these patients are also depressed. This mental state makes it extremely difficult for the patient to lose weight. These surgeons condemn these patients to be in chronic pain with all the complications related to a patient with chronic pain.

We, as physicians, should be able to recognize differences in culture and races. Patients interpret pain in different ways. There is a difference between magnification and maliciously fake pain. Overreaction is also a misinterpreted behavioral reaction. There is different emotional manifestation of pain in different races. Pain threshold and pain manifestation varies in each racial group. Pain expression and tolerance is also different between male and female. In my experience, I have seen patients fare better when they understand their condition and the physician takes the time to explain the possible causes of pain, their radiological studies, the anatomy of the spine, and some other issues related to LBP.

The medical information must be interpreted and taken with reservations. In fact, certain medical conditions have suffered a complete reversal on the treatment approach. For instance, years ago, the concept of bed rest for the first few days was widely accepted as a standard treatment of LBP in the medical community. People with LBP were advised to take bed rest for a few days and then resume regular duties. This is an extremely general concept. Now, it is recommended they continue regular duties without necessarily staying in bed for days.

I cannot overemphasize these statements: The same treatment cannot apply to all people with LBP. There are several causes of LBP. The treatment may vary from person to person with the same low back condition. The treatment has to be tailored to the person's constitution, age, habits, pain threshold, profession, and so forth. Therefore, reading common public literature about LBP should be taken with reservations.

The same treatment for the same condition can be given at different stages, times, and settings. A patient may feel more comfortable staying close to home for surgery, but other patients may feel safer having surgery at a large facility.

Treating a patient does not mean to prescribe a pill, do surgery, or please or fight an individual or insurance company. To treat a patient is to empathize, feel his or her concerns and worries, become part of his or her pain and frustrations (emphatic), and to be able to understand his or her nature. It is being able to choose the best treatment for this particular person and applying it to the individual's personality, physical demands (job), family needs, and psychological status.

The practice of medicine is a science and an art. When it comes to treating human beings, certain intuition and accurate common sense are needed. This art is not learned in a classroom nor is it taught by another colleague. The art of combining skills is an innate characteristic that physicians must have. It is something the physician will learn to recognize and perfect throughout years of practice and experience. It is a subtle, invisible force that some call intuition. This is the real medicine. A surgeon may possess the best skills, but he or she may have poor surgical and medical judgment and common sense. Medical schools do not train students to have common sense and instincts. These are the principles and pillars of EBM.

Most textbooks and journals recommend that primary care physicians refer patients to the spine specialist if they continue to have low back and leg pain after four or six weeks. After three months of leg pain due to a herniated disc, the chances for recovery after surgery may decrease. Plus, the chances for nerve damage increase. There are some exceptions to the rule of four to six weeks of conservative treatment for a patient with LBP and a disc herniation. These exceptions include cauda equina, progressive neurological deficits (numbness, weakness, absent reflexes on the exam, sphincter dysfunction), and severe leg pain.

Most medical textbooks and journals say that ninety percent of patients with sciatica or LBP will improve without surgery after one or two years. However, after four years, LBP recurs in as much as fifteen percent of patients. Therefore, the percentage of nonsurgical improvement for patients with a herniated disc falls from ninety percent to eighty-five prevent following these statistics. Fifteen percent of the patients will have chronic LBP, leg pain, and possibly nerve damage.

Physicians can become bitter due to ungrateful patients and the constantly changing health care system. Eager attorneys are waiting to destroy a physician's reputation and collect money. Some situations in the medical system can also alter medical judgment. The traps and other loopholes of the "every day more difficult health care system" cloud the physician's judgment.

The decisions for treatment may be biased. We, as physicians, must isolate these other factors and concentrate only on our patients' well-being. No good clinical judgment can be made with a clouded mind.

In my opinion, there is not necessarily a standard treatment for patients with low back conditions. Health insurance companies, HMOs, managed care, and others dictate standard regulations or rules for treatments.

We tend to follow advice that comes from reputable sources, but one must be cautious when interpreting data and recommendations from these sources. For instance, the source will say, "*All* patients with LBP will improve in time, and, with conservative treatment, only ten percent will require surgery." (Usually, publications mention this "rule" when referring only to patients with herniated discs in the lumbar spine.) In my opinion, this is a false statement, and the percentage is higher.

Patients, physicians, and insurance companies tend to make a "universal law" out of these concepts based on an isolated study that has no clear data collection. Most physicians and insurance companies use these concepts for the treatment and evaluation of patients with LBP.

Because general practitioners, physiatrists, occupational medicine physicians, and other physicians treat patients with surgical problems conservatively, they might endanger the patient's safety, increase the cost of treatment, and inflate the size of the health care system by following rigid guidelines or flowcharts. The patient (after delayed surgery) will need more postoperative care and rehabilitation, not to mention the legal implications of a delayed operation. The patient will also lose more time from work if surgery is delayed while waiting for or trying conservative treatment.

Who determines the surgical patient versus the nonsurgical patient? Spine surgeons ultimately will make a recommendation for or against surgery. A spine surgeon can compile information with a more complete global picture and a better understanding of the patient, and we can determine the necessity for surgery. We have a good idea of the prognosis based on global information pertaining to the patient with LBP. At the time of surgery, we see the extent of the injury. We learn to associate the clinical presentation with the radiological studies, surgical findings, recuperation, rehabilitation, and outcome. However, the treatment of a patient with LBP is generally a team approach that is coordinated by the primary care physician.

In the medical system, the primary care physician sees the patient with LBP first in order to initiate treatment before referring the patient to a spine surgeon. Occupational medicine physicians and chiropractors also see the patient beforehand. Now, there is a relatively new approach in which the patient is sent to a pain specialist. This approach (referring the patient to a pain specialist before sending the patient to a spine surgeon) originated from the idea that surgeons were abusing the system by performing too many unnecessary surgeries. However, there are more honest surgeons than dishonest ones.

Paradoxically, as one gains more experience and confidence while performing surgery, one (such as a spine surgeon) becomes more cautious and conservative when recommending surgery. Insurance companies sometimes believe they are saving money for the company by avoiding surgery when, in fact, it is the opposite in many situations.

Sometimes, the health care system may also be working in the opposite direction. By sending patients to a health care provider for primary, nonsurgical treatment, the system may spend more money than necessary because certain physicians may order studies that are not necessarily indicated in every case (for example, nerve tests, CT scans, discograms, and so forth). In some cases, conservative treatments such as steroid ("cortisone") injections, epidural shots, physical therapy, chiropractic treatments, and other alternative treatment procedures may create more expenses for the health care system than if surgery had been done at an earlier date.

It was not until recently that more reports were published in medical spine journals relating to the natural history of patients with disc herniation. These publications have finally recognized the necessity of classifying the patient with LBP, and they have specifically found that certain patients with herniated discs benefit more from early surgery than from conservative treatment. Not only does the patient benefit from early surgery (pain relief), but this form of treatment also saves the health care system huge amounts of money.

Primary care physicians follow guidelines or flowcharts for the treatment of a patient with LBP. They think that, by following these guidelines, they are helping patients and saving economic resources. The problem is that there are gaps in the interpretation of these guidelines.

In general, the best remedy for back pain is good physical condition and fitness, a regular program of exercise, good diet. Mostly, it is also avoiding postures, activities, and circumstances that trigger pain or cause more pain. One must recognize that some conditions have no cure, and one should avoid worsening of a condition. It is my observation that patients frequently look for solace and understanding. Patients also feel some level of comfort and even improvement when they can put a picture or image of their spinal condition in their brains. They can see the damage and on X-rays or an MRI scan. I like to explain to patients in detail the reading of an MRI scan. This practice helps a great deal for a better understanding of the patient, and their expectations are more realistic.

Example Cases

The following are four examples of treatment for different patients with LBP:

Example #1: Mr. John Doe, age thirty-five, after bending and lifting a piece of equipment at work, develops LBP without leg pain or neurological deficits (such as numbness, weakness, bladder or rectal dysfunction, decreased or absent reflexes) and has an otherwise unremarkable MRI scan. I would not recommend surgery. I would treat this patient conservatively. Most likely, he has only a muscle sprain/strain, facet joint pain, or some other benign, nonsurgical condition. If this patient undergoes surgery, the prognosis would be poor.

Example #2: Mr. John Doe, age forty-five, after doing heavy labor at work, develops low back and leg pain. The pain radiates into the posterior aspect of the left leg down to the level of the calf. He has tingling and numbness off and on. He sometimes feels weakness in the legs. He has no bladder or rectal difficulty. On exam, he has a decreased ankle reflex, and the numbness affects the lateral aspect of the calf and foot. He has a positive SLR on the left leg. He has LBP and leg pain constantly, and he cannot sleep due to the pain. He has more pain when standing and walking. Sitting also causes a great deal of pain after thirty minutes. The patient had physical therapy and has tried different pain medications and muscle relaxants for six weeks to no avail. The lumbar spine MRI scan shows a herniated disc and some degree of spinal stenosis at L4-5. This patient is married and still has children that require care and attention. He is active and wants to continue with a normal life.

He works as a supervisor and does some climbing, kneeling, and other chores considered as moderate work in his job. I do a thorough history and exam. I review the MRI scan with the patient and his wife and explain the spine anatomy and the MRI results. I give them some of the most current treatment options and discuss surgery, which I strongly recommend to avoid permanent nerve damage. Surgery would also bring him back into a normal life and avoid prolonged work absence. Inactivity and prolonged work absence may cause depression and frustration that will affect the patient so much that, by the time he has surgery (if delayed), the patient will be more difficult to deal with. He will have a longer recovery, and the success rate may drop, regardless of the surgical technique utilized. I would mention alternatives to surgery such as epidural blocks (controversial) and endoscopic surgery. If the disc herniation is too large by MRI scan, an endoscopic procedure may not be suitable for the patient. Other alternatives such as IDET, nucleoplasty, and so forth are a consideration. But, if the disc is large, I doubt the disc herniation will resolve with these techniques.

The patient must take part in the decision-making process on the type of surgical technique to be used. However, I still maintain my recommendations as a surgeon. I would recommend a microdisketomy with no fusion. Recent studies favor early surgery when indicated. It has been concluded that early surgery may not only improve the patient's symptoms and misery, but also control cost by decreasing loss of working days, early rehabilitation, and less chances for developing chronic pain, depression, drug addiction, and, in general, poor response to late surgery. The longer a patient stays out of work, the less chances of ever returning to work. This behavior and pattern has been observed in different studies.

Notice the level of the disc herniation and spinal stenosis is at L4-5 (narrow spinal canal) and there are some other factors for which I would consider surgery on this specific patient. However, if the disc herniation was at L5-S1, my recommendations might be less invasive, and I would possibly suggest trying more conservative treatment for four weeks before surgery was warranted. This recommendation would only be if the patient has no serious neurological deficits, is still walking, and is carrying on his ADLs.

There can be several variants in the treatment of this patient. Depending on the degree of herniation, the location of the herniated fragment, whether there is a free fragment, the size of the patient, and other considerations have to be taken into account.

This can be a controversial decision for surgery on this patient among surgeons and between clinicians and surgeons. Some spine surgeons may recommend a spinal fusion; others may suggest an endoscopic diskectomy.

Other surgeons would recommend a laser endoscopic surgery. If the disc is "small" according to the MRI scan, some may even recommend an IDET procedure. Some spine surgeons may require a "discogram" to decide on the use of spinal instrumentation and hardware for a fusion.

There are different approaches for the same condition. Depending on the patient's conditions, the surgeon's experience, and the underlying spine condition, one selects a specific surgical technique.

Example #3: Jane Doe, forty years of age, after getting up in the morning, develops severe LBP, numbness, and weakness in the legs. She has increasingly difficulty urinating and has not had a bowel movement in three days. The patient can barely stand and walk. On the exam, this patient has numbness, weakness, and severe low back and leg pain. There is a positive SLR. An MRI scan shows a large (massive) herniated disc with nerve impingement. There is no evidence of instability on the radiological studies. The patient goes to the local emergency room because she suddenly could not urinate anymore and had numbness in the genital region. I would recommend emergency surgery with a diskectomy and decompression (laminectomy) with no fusion.

Example #4: Jane Doe, fifty years of age, presents with severe LBP with radiation into the posterior aspect of the hips and down the leg to the foot. She has had numbness and (possibly) weakness in both legs. She has had chronic LBP for several years. Most recently, the pain has gotten worse. On the exam, the patient has a decreased ankle reflex on both sides, positive SLR, and decreased strength and sensation on both legs. The regular X-rays and MRI scan show a dislocation of L5-S1 (Spondylolisthesis grade III) with DDD and a protruding disc at the same level. She has used a back brace, has had extensive physical therapy, and has had two epidural blocks. She did not improve with any of these techniques of conservative and semiconservative treatment. She would not be a candidate for an IDET, epidural blocks, or any other semiconservative, invasive procedure. She will be a surgical candidate for a spinal fusion at L5-S1, provided she is medically stable and suitable for surgery.

CHAPTER 7

Health Insurance Systems

A Brief Explanation of How a Medical Office Works (Visiting the Physician)

Medical offices, hospitals, and other health care providers have to comply with rules and regulations established by state and federal laws. The Health Insurance Portability and Accountability Act (HIPAA) has recently established more new rules and has enforced old ones. HIPAA is directly related to the Secretary of Health and Human Services. Physicians and hospitals have to comply with HIPAA regulations. More information on these topics can be found in the appropriate sources. Books have been written about the evolving field of medical office management. New regulations related to this field develop every year. During the last twenty years, administrative medicine has transformed significantly. There are seminars, courses, books, audiotapes, and videotapes that teach how to make a medical office work more efficiently and how to comply with federal and state laws. There are also courses for secretaries to teach them about front desk, billing and collections, and office management.

Medical offices usually have a staff that involves the following:

- Office manager
- Front desk secretary or receptionist
- A billing and collections clerk. (There may be one for billing and one for collections.) Sometimes, physicians' offices use a collection agency.
- Transcription secretaries or agencies that do medical transcriptions
- Filing clerk
- Coding clerk

Some physicians' offices have only one, two, or more employees for the above functions. Each medical practice is different. Most insurance companies require the physician's office staff to submit a billing claim in order to be paid.

Special computer programs are utilized in medical offices. The principle of these computer programs is to use office resources in a more productive, efficient, and economical manner.

Usually, the front desk receptionist greets the patient and obtains personal information. The patient is typically asked to fill out paperwork with personal and insurance information. Copies of a driver's license or other documents may be required during the registration process. All of this information is confidential. If the patient refuses to fill out the required information, the physician's manager will try to solve any possible conflict. The appointment might have to be rescheduled until the conflict is resolved.

Each physician has his or her own system. Rules and policies of a medical office are usually posted in the office waiting room. The patient should be aware of the most important office policies.

Some physicians have the patient file his or her insurance claim. Some physician's office staff may ask for payment in advance before the medical service is rendered. However, most physicians (as a service to the patient) will bill the insurance company. In many instances, patients ignore the billing and collections processes. Sometimes, billing and collections is made through the hospital, medical associations such as an IPA, or other medical associations ("clearinghouse" companies). Some offices accept credit cards, and others do not take personal checks.

Most physicians have an office manager who coordinates and supervises all office personnel. The office manager is generally trained in all areas of a medical office, such as front desk, office policies, billing and collections, and other tasks.

Each person in a medical office has job descriptions. For instance, a front desk receptionist typically takes telephone calls, relays messages, makes appointments, sets up studies, and fills prescriptions with the physician's authorization.

The person in charge of billing and collections will usually deal with coding and insurance companies. He or she will also assist patients with insurance claims and financial arrangements. Most physicians' offices customarily file the claims to insurance companies as a courtesy, but physicians are not necessarily obligated to do this work. It is ultimately the patient's responsibility to have claims submitted and paid. Physicians may have a contract with an insurance company that requires them to file billing claims. Some offices use an external billing or collections agency or contract with a company often from out of town.

Sometimes, confusion occurs between patients and the physician's office personnel. When there are administrative and financial conflicts, they may turn into unpleasant situations for both the patient and the physician. Patients assume the physician's office will do all the administrative paperwork and that it will be performed accurately.

Most physicians will accept to see patients with no health insurance; however, conflicts arise due to lack of communication. The office manager or billing and collections clerk may work a financial arrangement to make payments more convenient to the patient's income schedule. It is relatively common that patients deceive the physician's office staff with false financial information for not having an economic status that allows them to cover their debts and for fear of not being seen. A deceitful patient might make a physician terminate a physician-patient relationship.

Usually a primary care physician refers a patient to another physician or facility for consultations. Insurance companies may need the primary care physician to make referrals to a specialist instead of referring patients from specialist to specialist. Sometimes, the insurance company may not need the patient to be referred by a primary care physician to a specialist. The insurance may let the patient see a specialist without a referral.

Physicians have the right to choose which patients to see and which insurance plans to accept in the office. For instance, a physician may not want to see patients with Medicaid and/or Medicare. Doctors have the freedom to contract with health insurance companies (and become a provider of the company). The patient should check with the insurance if a particular study or procedure was authorized before it is done. I recommend, when contacting an insurance company, getting the person's name that authorized the procedure, the date and time of the call, and telephone numbers.

Sometimes, physician's offices have consent forms for surgical procedures that patients are required to sign before surgery. Occasionally, patients become frustrated by the paperwork they have to fill out, especially the elderly that often have difficulty reading the questions or do not understand the policies and insurance jargon. Some offices have secretaries to assist patients in filling out these forms. It is very important that all information contained in any form filled out and signed in the physician's office is accurate.

Normally, health insurance companies provide a card with important rules written on the back of the card. There are phone numbers to call for information and notification if the patient is using the services of the insurance. The doctor's secretary may make a copy of the card for further reference. The doctor's secretary may also call to verify eligibility and notify the insurance carrier of the doctor's visit. When there is a medical emergency, many insurance companies give twenty-four to forty-eight hours to notify them of the medical emergency. Some insurance companies will not cover expenses if they are not notified of an emergency admission if the patient or his or her relatives did not follow the insurance's rules.

The Health Insurance Systems and Medical Coverage

There are several types of health care insurance or medical coverage for sickness or accident-related injuries. There are also some forms of disability that cover medical expenses and compensation for losses due to inability to work. The Americans with Disabilities Act (ADA) ensures that employers will treat Americans fairly when patients have certain disabilities. If interested in learning more about it, I recommend getting further information related to ADA from the appropriate sources. The Family and Medical Leave Act (FMLA) (U.S. Department of Labor) addresses maintenance of health insurance by an employer when under a group health plan. Specifically, under FMLA, a job position must be kept open for a person that needs to take time off from work (usually about twelve weeks) due to either sickness or injury for the employee or a close family member.

This is a summary of the most common types of medical coverage:

- Private insurance that can be acquired through an employer or individually
- Commercial insurance companies
- HMO (Health Maintenance Organization)
- PPO (Preferred Provider Organization)
- MHO (Medical-Hospital Organization)
- Workers' compensation
- Medicare
- Medicaid
- Auto insurance
- DVR (Division of Vocational Rehabilitation)
- Community and nonprofit organizations and clinics
- Regional or state clinics
- University hospitals
- VA (Veterans Administration) and military health institutions
- Private pay or self-pay
- Indigent funds (county, state, and so forth)
- Federal Employers Liability Act (FELA)

- Federal Employees' Compensation Act (FECA)
- Longhorn & Harbor Workers Compensation Act
- Merchant Marine Act
- Office of Workers' Compensation Program (OWCP). (This office involves some of the above types of federal employees' compensation.)
- Indian medical services
- Other

Medicare. Most people are familiar with the Medicare and Medicaid systems. However, I will briefly mention how they work. The government typically provides Medicare to people older than sixty-five. However, people with permanent injuries or disabilities can sometimes qualify for Medicare. When under Medicare coverage, there is no need for authorization for studies or surgery, but it has some restriction on coverage for medical supplies, prescriptions, home health care, physical therapy, dental, and corrective eyeglasses. People need to qualify for Medicare under government rules.

There are some states in which Medicaid became part of an HMO and functions in a similar manner. Authorization is required for certain studies, emergency room and doctor's office visits, surgery, and so forth. They function as any other private health insurance.

Medicare covers medical costs just as a commercial insurance would for health-related conditions. Patients should be aware of these rules and regulations. A physician may elect whether or not to be a Medicare or Medicaid provider. Physicians who participate take "assignment." This means the physician agrees to be paid only the allowable fee, which can be as low as twenty percent of the regular physician's fees. Medicare pays eighty percent of the allowable. The other twenty percent is collected from the patient. If there is a secondary supplemental health insurance, this other insurance pays the other twenty percent of the total bill. If the physician does not take assignment, the physician is entitled to charge the patient the remainder of the outstanding balance (that is, his or her regular fee).

Medicaid. Medicaid is similar to Medicare. Medicaid covers medical expenses for people with low income and a certain number of family (children) members. Sometimes, children qualify for Medicaid but not their parents.

VAH (Veteran Administration Hospital) is another medical service provided for government employees and veterans. They also have their own rules.

There are different ways that physicians charge their fees for service. Most will charge for the deductible if not met during the year, or they may charge the "copay" or both. How does a physician set his or her fees? Some people ask this question. Typically, there are several factors that insurance companies and medical associations consider to set physician's fees. Several years ago, there were no HMOs dictating physician's fees. Medical associations and physicians set their own fees. Insurance companies paid one hundred percent of those fees without much questioning. There are medical associations and specialty associations that usually have a standard fee schedule.

Currently, medical associations and insurance companies work hand in hand to set those fees. However, as medical competition has increased, physicians accept lower fees. In other words, it is now up to the HMOs and insurance companies to pay only "customary fees."

It is not my intention with this book to delve into all forms of health insurance rules and polices. I suggest reading appropriate books related to these topics. However, I think it will be worthwhile to outline and overview some specific forms of medical coverage such as workers' compensation.

The Workers' Compensation System

I will make general comments about the workers' compensation system. I do not intend to cover all aspect of this extensive field. I do not consider myself an expert in this area. I think people should have basic information about health care systems and compensation insurance companies. I am continuously asked about medical coverage and workers' compensation.

Workers' compensation is an insurance that covers mainly medical expenses for injuries or illness arising from work-related accident and exposure. In some instances, workers' compensation also covers compensations when there is less income or no income at all. By state law, most employers must provide workers' compensation insurance for their employees. Sometimes, the employers have a contract with an insurance company. Others may have subcontractors, or employers may have their own medical coverage.

According to the legislation of the state, some employers must provide workers' compensation insurance for on-the-job injuries and illness that resulted from exposure at work. The Workers' Compensation Act does not apply to employers in farm and ranch operations in the state of New Mexico (McKinney v. Davis, 84 N.M. 352, 503 P.2d 332,1972). Therefore, when employees sustain an injury at work while working on a farm in the state of New Mexico, the employee has no medical coverage. Many times, these employees do not have regular health insurance either. They apply for Medicaid or Medicare, and they are sometimes denied.

There are states in which workers' compensation has the Division of Vocational Rehabilitation (DVR), an area of workers' compensation designed to retrain employees when necessary. Some other times, DVR is independent of workers' compensation and is run by the state.

Usually, the employee is required to fill out an incident or accident report after any work-related injury. This accident or incident report is very important. The more detailed the report, the better it is to prove later the extent of injuries and the body part involved. This report is also very important to explain and determine the extent of the injuries.

Different workers' compensation companies also have different policies and regulations that must be followed. They have their own list of medical conditions covered, and their own system of assessing the injured person. (Sometimes, they have what is called a "schedule" of medical conditions.) They have a medical diagnosis for injury to certain body parts that already have certain percentage of impairment and compensation. The insurance personnel typically investigate the case until they decide if there has been a work-related injury and if it will cover medical expenses.

Some insurance companies have a list of providers. Some companies will let the employee select any physician for evaluation and treatment during the first thirty, sixty, or ninety days after a work-related injury. After that time, the insurance has the right to send the patient to one of its health care providers for further evaluation and treatment. However, the patient still has the right to choose treatment among the choices given by the physician. The patient can also choose his or her own surgeon if surgery is required or recommended.

The patient should not be obligated to see a specific surgeon, to have surgery with a specific surgeon, or to have a specific treatment. However, if the patient refuses the treatment recommended by a physician, the insurance might have the right to terminate medical coverage. Insurance companies usually have the right to stop compensation and medical care if the patient does not comply or abide by the treating physician's recommendations.

When there is a dispute between a patient and an insurance company, attorneys may be involved, and they may ask the treating physicians to appear for depositions for a medical opinion. They may hire certain physicians as expert witnesses. Usually, a person from the insurance company is assigned by the company to deal directly with the worker. These persons are called adjusters or case managers. Sometimes, these persons have some medical background (nurses) with a master's degree in science or administration. I will answer some of the most common questions related to this topic at the end of this chapter. Sometimes, there is the need of "mediation" to come to an agreement between employer and employee about covering for expenses incurred in work-related injuries.

Fraud. There are states in which malingering is considered as fraud and a felony, and the employee can be penalized. Patients faking an injury are called "malingerers" in medicine. It is not unusual that a patient magnifies symptoms to seek disability. There is a difference between the patient who has no objective evidence of an injury (with normal X-rays, MRI scan, CT scan, and so forth) and complains of pain and the patients with proven injuries (objectively proven by medical exam and studies).

There are patients that do have medical evidence of injuries, but the patient magnifies or exaggerates symptoms. These are probably the most common groups of patients. These patients are hard to manage medically and difficult to handle for disability. Many of these patients have secondary gains that can be monetary, psychological, or both. They usually are chronic complainers. They can have a litigious personality who will seek legal action against all professional people involved with them. These patients also alter data.

Patients can respond in any of the following ways to a work-related injury:

- The legitimately injured patient. The patient does not exhibit signs of magnification, emotional overreaction, or malingering.

- Magnification and exaggeration of symptoms (consciously or unconsciously). Patients sometimes get hurt at work because of their animosity against the employer or against the type of job they do (job dissatisfaction). Other times, employees get hurt because they are tired ("burnt out") of doing the same job for several years or because they look for a way out (consciously or unconsciously). They look for an excuse to retire.

- Overreaction. There are patients who are very emotional and overreact to pain.

- Anger/Frustration/Depression. Patients fall in the vicious cycle of frustration-anger-depression-anxiety-more pain. These patients are difficult to treat medically. Some of these patients also react with anger and resentment against employers and health providers. Some of these complaints may or may not be legitimate. Sometimes, these patients are treated with certain disdain because physicians and insurance companies suspect malingering. The lack of understanding of their problems generates more anger and the need for legal action.

- Malingering. This involves faking an injury for secondary gains.

All these situations and responses make some physicians uncomfortable handling patients with work-related injuries. These patients frequently involve physicians in legal processes that are not only time-consuming for the health care providers, but they are also stressful for the physician. These proceedings may pose legal risks for the professional involved in litigation cases. However, following medical and ethical standards, one, as a physician, should be able to deal with these patients and their insurance companies. Not all physicians are familiar with the workers' compensation systems, jargon, and terms. Not all physicians are familiar with the medical evaluation of these patients (Impairment Rating, Independent Medical Evaluation, and so forth).

The Degenerative Spine and the Preexisting Medical Condition. Most workers' compensation (federal) agencies recognize that most adults have some degree of degenerative changes in the spine (joints and bone) as part of the aging process. Therefore, the person who sustains a work-related injury (back injury) should have some type of medical coverage provided by the employer; however, each state has its own rules and regulations. Accidents might aggravate or exacerbate a previous medical condition as we see on MRI scan studies. It is possible to sustain a new injury that can be found on diagnostic studies. For the physician, there are clues when reading a spinal MRI scan to know whether an injury is new or is an aggravation of a previous one. The majority of patients I see in my office after a work-related injury have already some degree of spinal deterioration, degenerative disc disease, spondylosis ("arthritis"), bulging discs, spinal stenosis, and so forth. An injury or exposure can aggravate, exacerbate, precipitate, or accelerate lower back conditions. A medical condition can occur related to certain exposures or accidents, and one, as a physician, must give an opinion on probability and possibility. Probability is when there is more than a fifty percent chance that an exposure or injury would be related to a certain outcome. Possibility is when there is less than a fifty percent chance of correlation between injury (or exposure) and outcome.

These are some of the most common terms used in the workers' compensation setting in a medical evaluation:

- Aggravation is when a previous medical condition becomes permanently worse due to accident or exposure to an agent.

- Exacerbation is the same definition as above, except the medical condition becomes worse only temporarily.

- Acceleration is when a medical condition would have manifest in time, but exposure to an agent made it appear sooner.

- Recurrence is the appearance of symptoms without a triggering accident or exposure and is related to a previous injury or illness.

- Precipitation is when an agent makes a smoldering process appear or manifest its symptoms and signs.

There are subsets of variants in this arena, such as the case when an employee has a previous medical condition (prior to a work-related accident or exposure). For instance, a patient has a seizure (epilepsy) and has a head injury at work. Should the accident account for all work-related injuries and the medical condition in this person? There is a situation in medicine that is called *apportionment* in which a physician determines and *allocates* certain injuries to the preexisting condition and other percentage of the injuries or allocation is given to the patient because of work-related injuries. Most workers' compensation insurance companies will cover medical expenses for injuries or diseases that are directly related to an accident or exposure at work, regardless of the so-called "preexisting condition."

Most workers' compensation insurance companies cover medical expenses for injuries and illnesses for life. For instance, if an employee sustains an injury or an illness occur at a certain job and the employee changes jobs later on, if the employee sustained another injury or illness (at the same anatomical body part or body system) at the new job, the first employer might be liable still for the injuries. But, if there is a new injury or illness not closely related to the first one, the current employer is liable. If a patient has a ruptured disc at L4-5 at one job and the employee now ruptures L5-S1 at a second job, the second employer is liable for the new injury (L5-S1) but not for the previous one (L4-5). However, one must remember that each state has different laws and regulations.

Motor Vehicle Accident/Motor Vehicle Collision (MVA/MVC)

There are different types of medical coverage. Patients usually are covered for medical coverage, but there is a limit on the payment by the insurance. Some physicians avoid seeing patients that have been involved in car accidents because of the legal implication. These patients become a challenge for the physician, and they are difficult to treat because of the multiple complaints and the lack of improvement with any treatment (secondary gain). It is frustrating for a physician to treat these patients. Few physicians are familiar with the legal jargon and terms involved with cases that involve attorneys and judges.

There are physicians who devote their time for medical testimony after being trained formally as "expert witnesses." Directories and lists of "expert witnesses" are available for attorneys.

Social Security/Disability

Government agencies determine disability based on certain rules. The physician provides government agencies with copies of medical records upon a formal request from the patient or attorney. There are physicians who specialize in disability evaluations and provide government agencies and attorneys with copies of medical records. Sometimes, there is a need for a special medical evaluation that follows a written report by a physician. The physician makes recommendations in the report, but the decision for disability (and the type of disability) depends on the government agencies and judges. A patient might be disabled for certain activities but not for others. It is rare when a person qualifies for total permanent disability. Not all physicians are familiar with the process of disability reports and filling out disability forms. For disability determination, there is no need to have a percentage of impairment in a medical evaluation report, as is the case in workers' compensation.

I suggest consulting appropriate literature and books such as the American Medical Association and the "Guides to the Evaluation of Permanent Impairment" to find the definition of disability, impairment, handicap, and so forth. I will briefly mention some of these definitions and topics in the questions at the end of this chapter.

Medical Diagnostic and Procedural Coding

Coding is a system created relatively recently, and it has gradually become more complicated. Physicians and insurance companies are constantly trying to find methods to make this administrative process more efficient, but these systems sometimes work against physicians, insurance companies, and patients. The more complex the billing system, the more need for personnel that require appropriate training (more expenses). It is difficult to find experienced personnel in this area. The basis of this coding system for medical diagnosis and treatments is that insurance companies will have better control of medical services and billing practices. There are two basic coding systems:

- **CPT:** Current Procedural Terminology
- **ICD-9:** International Classification of Diseases (9th Revision) or Index of Coding Diagnosis

There are different techniques to code a medical diagnostic procedure. Some of the main coding books are CPT, ICD-9, McGraw-Hill, Anthony's, and others. Most insurance companies, including Medicare and Medicaid, use these codes.

Sometimes, one person in a physician's office is strictly in charge of medical coding. This person should have specific training just for coding. ICD-9 and CPT books provide a specific number for each diagnosis and for each medical procedure respectively. For instance, for a disc herniation in the lower back, there is an ICD-9 number or code, 722.10. This number is very important when filling out and filing a medical claim. This is the number that gives the insurance company a diagnosis and for which the physician is billing a charge.

The CPT number code is a medical procedure number. Surgery, injections, and any invasive procedure or service rendered in the office or on an outpatient or inpatient basis have a specific CPT code number. For instance, for an L4-5 discectomy, there is a CPT code number, 63030. Services such as consultations, advice, opinions, and so forth also involve a CPT code. Hospitals may use a different coding system to bill insurance companies.

Most insurance companies require both the CPT and the ICD-9 coding numbers. Coding could be a little more complicated. The CPT and the ICD-9 codes have to match in a claim for the insurance company to pay a bill. Even physicians have to take workshops, seminars, and courses to learn appropriate ways of coding procedures.

There are special courses, training, and books for health insurance companies, medical practice management, billing, collections, front desk, coding, medical associations, medical rules and regulations, workers' compensation, and so forth. I recommend consulting the appropriate sources for this information because I have outlined only some of the principles and simple systems related to medical offices, hospitals, and so forth.

Questions

I dedicate this section mainly to workers' compensation patients. These are some of the most frequent questions patients ask me.

What do I do after I have been hurt at work? Depending on the severity of the injury, the patient may be taken to an emergency department or a clinic specializing in occupational medicine for evaluation and treatment. It is beneficial for the patient or his or her family members to obtain the medical report of the accident and the extent of the injuries from the emergency room physician.

What is an incident or accident report? An incident or accident report is an important form that employers have. This form or report is required to use as a proof of the on-the-job injury or illness. This form will be used by workers' compensation to determine medical coverage. It is recommended completing the report or form soon after the accident. Witnesses of the accident are also important to add further proof of the accident at work. I recommend getting names of witnesses, addresses, phone numbers, and so forth. It is recommended documenting the date and details of the accident accurately. If the employer sent the employee to a specific health provider such as a chiropractor, it should be mentioned in the report. If the employer orders the employee to continue working, it will be advisable to mention that in the report. This initial report is very important for future claims and for legal purposes.

When can I go back to work? This is a rather broad question with different answers. That depends on the type of work the person performs and on the kind of injury the worker sustained. There are guidelines in special books to this matter. Some books contain statistics on the time it takes workers to return to work depending on the type of injury. These books precisely guide the practitioner on when a worker can return to work. However, the final decision for return to work depends on the treating physician. Sometimes, the physician may recommend the patient do not return to heavy work. Light duty might be permitted for the employee. The employee might be totally disabled for the regular job the employee has performed, but not for other positions. I will not impose any return to work time frame in this book after a work-related injury. I have my own opinion, but my practice may be controversial to other physicians and employers. Is an employee at the risk for reinjury if he or she is sent back to work prematurely? That depends on how we define prematurely. A patient may be able to go back to work in a couple of days if the injury was a simple strain or sprain.

What is a reasonable time for an employee to heal from a back condition after an injury? To answer this question, it will be necessary to know the type of injury the patient sustained and the kind of work the employee performs. It varies, for instance, for a sprain/strain. The employee may be taking off work anywhere from just a couple of days to a couple of weeks. For an employee who underwent back surgery, it depends on the type of surgery the patient underwent, but the time to heal, recover, and rehabilitate after surgery may be anywhere between 70 and 140 days (nonfusion and fusion surgery). This decision is to be made by the treating surgeon using basic medical knowledge and common sense and abiding by some guidelines established in certain books.

What kind of work status should I be placed on after I sustained a work-related injury? Work status is usually determined by the physician involved in the care of a patient who has been involved in a work-related injury. Physicians who specialize in industrial or occupational medicine usually have the experience to treat patients for work-related injuries and are able to interact with workers' compensation and other insurance companies.

Who determines work status, impairment rating, disability, and return to work date? An occupational medicine physician can fill out a specific request from workers' compensation addressing work status, physical limitations, diagnosis, estimated return to work time, and permanent or temporary physical limitations and capabilities. Special reports or medical evaluations are required by employers in some instances to relocate or accept the employee back to work. If the injury involves only a strain, sprain, or a minor injury or if the patient was treated and healed completely for a medical condition, it is likely the worker will not have a permanent disability. The employee can return to work without physical restrictions after a reasonable and customary period of treatment. If the patient had surgery, the surgeon can also give an impairment rating, disability, work status, and so forth. However, a primary care physician and/or an occupational medicine physician should be able to evaluate a patient even after surgery. When an Independent Medical Evaluation (IME) is requested, it must be performed by other than the treating physicians. Usually special training is required to learn to use the AMA *Guides to the Evaluation of Permanent Impairment*. Special courses and seminars are offered to obtain certification as an IME, disability and IR evaluator.

On the other hand, a patient may be disabled from his or her job, but not necessarily for a different type of work. This situation frequently gets confusing for patients because they expect one hundred percent or complete disability due to their injuries. However, a patient may be disabled one hundred percent for his or her former job (for instance, heavy work), but he or she may be able to perform light or sedentary duties. Depending on the job description and activities that are required to carry out the job, the patient may or may not be one hundred percent disabled. Partial or temporary disability may apply in particular situations. Most frequently, after a work-related injury, a patient is placed on these are the work capacities.

A patient may be on temporary or permanent disability; at the same time, a patient can be:

- **Fully disabled** for any kind of work or for the work the employee was performing at the time of the injury. However, a patient can be disabled for heavy work but not for other types of work such as sedentary or light duty.

- **Partially disabled.** This disability can be temporary or permanent.

Work categories and capacities tend to be standard. They can vary from state to state, but there are generally four categories:

- **Sedentary Work.** This involves occasional lifting a maximum of ten pounds. Walking and standing are occasional in sedentary work (for instance, office work).

- **Light Work.** This involves lifting only up to a maximum of twenty pounds with frequent lifting and carrying of objects weighing up to ten pounds. In this work, standing and walking are required to a significant extent. There is also sitting, pushing, and pulling and a use of arms and legs to a certain degree. Light work can be subdivided into Light Medium Work in which the lifting limitation is thirty pounds with occasional and frequent lifting or carrying objects up to twenty pounds.

- **Moderate or Medium Work.** The weight lifting maximum is fifty pounds and frequent lifting and carrying up to twenty-five pounds.

- **Heavy work.** Light Heavy Work involves lifting up to seventy-five pounds and frequent lifting and carrying up to forty pounds. Heavy Work allows one hundred pounds as maximum lifting. Frequent carrying and lifting fifty pounds are allowed.

When a physician performs an evaluation for disability, several factors are taken into consideration: previous injuries, associated injuries or extensiveness of injuries or previous medical conditions, previous back injuries and other spine disorders associated with a disc herniation (for instance, spinal stenosis), the type of work the employee performs, the age of the patient, and so forth. A physician determines what work category the worker can perform. Occasionally, a Functional Capacity Evaluation (FCE) is performed to get guidelines for physical limitations. An FCE can be ordered by the treating physician, the evaluating physician, the workers' compensation adjuster, or the attorneys involved in a case.

I evaluate patients for impairment and disability by following guidelines set forth in appropriate resources and textbooks and using medical logistics and common sense (EBM). If there is a patient with a lumbar disc herniation for which the patient requires surgery (and undergoes an operation), I usually abide by the AMA *Guides to the Evaluation of Permanent Impairment* to set an impairment rating. I also recommend physical limitations mostly for bending, stooping, and lifting. There is controversy on weight lifting limitations for patients with low back injuries, but, in general, if a patient has a disc herniation(s) with or without surgery, I arbitrarily recommend lifting occasionally only up to thirty-five pounds, avoiding twisting and bending the lower back, avoiding rides in bumpy vehicles, standing and walking for prolonged periods, stooping, kneeling, and crawling. If the patient has neurological impairment such as numbness or weakness in the legs, I provide other physical limitations. I recommend these patients avoid climbing stairs and ladders and sitting or driving for prolonged periods in some cases (truck drivers). By prolonged sitting, standing, and walking, I mean activities that require more than four continuous hours in one day in an eight-hour shift. However, prolonged, limited, and restricted activities are terms than can be vague, and physicians can give different (personal) interpretations.

I usually discuss physical limitations, body mechanics, and ergonomics with the patient. If the patient is young and motivated to go back to work, I recommend the patient return to work in a regular capacity, but with precautions when performing moderate or heavy work. I recommend using body mechanics when working in general, especially after a patient had a back injury. Depending on the patient's job, physical structure, and other factors, restrictions may vary. There may be difference of opinions among physicians in their recommendations for physical restrictions and capabilities. I suggest getting an FCE sometimes for an objective physical evaluation on capabilities and limitations. I suggest patients consider retraining for a new job by institutions such as the Division of Vocational Rehabilitation (DVR) after a work-related injury has occurred and if the patient has a permanent impairment and there are physical restrictions for heavy work.

Physical capabilities and limitations on an injured patient can be controversial among physicians. Again, physical condition, age, gender, and other factors play an important role when determining physical limitations and impairment. There are physicians that do not set any physical limitations or provide any impairment to injured patients. Some states do not penalize physicians for returning employees to their former jobs.

Some scientific articles state a patient who had low back surgery or had a lumbar disc herniation should not necessarily avoid lifting objects. However, there is consensus in the medical community and within scientific papers that twisting (torque force) has a harmful effect on the spine and this activity should be restricted.

To my knowledge, there is no clear scientific data related to restrictions on physical activities on patients with a lumbar disc herniation (with and without surgery). It would be difficult to set physical limitations because every patient has a different physical structure and predisposition for injuries. Other factors can vary the response of the body to certain physical activities.

Physical limitations and impairment can be relative because a person may be disabled now, but, in six, twelve, or twenty-four months, the values of impairment rating and physical limitations may change. It is up to the insurance company to periodically repeat an impairment rating or medical evaluation for physical limitations and capabilities. The impairment and disability initially found on an evaluation may change with time as the patient evolves. Usually, the patient improves. However, the patient can also have a relapse. Some insurance companies request evaluations every six or twelve months.

Nevertheless, evaluations can be performed even after several years of the initial on-the-job injury.

I recommend individuals avoid bending, lifting, twisting, and prolonged sitting and standing. This advice is not only for the patient with a lower back condition or someone who has had back surgery, but also for the person with no symptoms of lower back problems. Anticipation and prevention are the best defense against wear and tear. Fortunately, there are ways to prolong this process. We must bear in mind that it has not been proven scientifically and conclusively that some of the above factors, such as obesity, smoking, bending, lifting, and sitting, will make the spine deteriorate.

What is *prolonged* sitting and standing? There is not a clear definition, but my theory is that sitting and standing straight for eight hours a day may eventually increase the chances of spinal deterioration. I recommend that, during an eight-hour shift, one should change positions from sitting to standing and walking. More details are given in the chapter on physical activities and posture. Cross-training and job rotation might help the employee and the employer to have a healthier and friendlier environment and relationship. Work can be more productive and efficient with these modifications or implementations.

If I am treating someone diagnosed with a herniated disc, physical restrictions might not be necessarily permanent. If the person has only a strain or a sprain, I still recommend that bending, twisting, and lifting objects over fifteen pounds should be discontinued during the recovery time. The lifting limitations can be controversial in some publications because it has not been conclusively established that lifting increases the chances for low back injuries. In fact, it is not only the act of lifting, but also the manner of lifting that can injure the lower back. One can injure the lower back by lifting only five or ten pounds; in contrast, one can move or lift as much as 100 pounds without injury if using proper body mechanics.

Who is a workers' compensation adjuster? An adjuster is usually the person assigned to a case by the insurance company (workers' compensation). Usually, the adjuster is in contact with the employee on a regular basis. The adjuster will guide the worker with instructions to follow for medical care and for other issues related to compensation. Sometimes, a case manager is also involved in a case. The person in charge is usually a nurse or someone with some medical background. This person and/or adjuster will coordinate appointments with physicians. Sometimes, the case manager accompanies the patient to the physician's office. The adjuster may or may not have medical background.

Will I need treatment for life? A worker will not necessarily need medical care for life. Some states mandate lifetime medical care for an injured worker. Other times, the insurance companies offer the employee a settlement.

Do I need an attorney? Patients may wonder if they need an attorney to deal with his or her insurance company. It is up to the patient whether to hire a lawyer or not. I do not interfere with the decision of the patient.

What is an MMI in the workers' compensation setting? MMI stands for maximum medical improvement. When (medically speaking) one expects no significant change in a medical condition in the next twelve months, one can say a patient has reached MMI. The medical condition has stabilized, and it is not likely to change with or without medical treatment. One, as a physician, expects no recovery or deterioration of the condition. However, some changes may still happen over time. The patient reaches a plateau in which a medical condition has stabilized. If a patient declines certain forms of treatment, such as surgery, injections, and so forth, the physician can place the worker at MMI.

Once the patient has reached MMI, the treating surgeon (if surgery was performed) usually releases the patient from his or her care to go back to the primary care physician. The surgeon releases the patient with some kind of work status and physical limitations, if applicable. The patient at this point is ready for an impairment rating for the injuries sustained at work. The patient can even have an IME if requested by any of the parties involved in the case.

What are the rules and regulations of the state workers' compensation? Each state has its set of rules and regulations. This information can be obtained from state institutions and agencies. There are also federal workers' compensation laws.

Do I need a second surgical opinion? Many insurance companies will not approve a surgical procedure without a second surgical opinion. If the physician performing a second surgical opinion disagrees with the first surgeon, there can be a third surgical opinion. The second surgical opinion surgeon may not agree with the first surgeon. It will be up to the patient, insurance companies, and attorneys (if involved) to follow the first or the second surgeon's advice. Another specialist of the same field usually performs a second opinion.

Who decides if a second surgical opinion is in order?

- The patient
- The insurance company
- The treating physician and/or the initial surgeon
- An attorney

The patient or the insurance company may choose the physician for a second surgical opinion, depending on the insurance benefits and policies. The same applies for other treatments, such as physical therapy, rehabilitation, orthopedic devices, speech therapy, and so forth. It is up to the patient's confidence in the surgeon whether to request a second surgical opinion or not. If the primary care physician disagrees with the surgeon, he or she can also request a second surgical opinion. If there are different surgical techniques that can be applied to the same patient, a surgeon may refer the patient to another surgeon for another opinion. The primary care physician also plays a role in the decision for a second surgical opinion.

One must bear in mind that patients sometimes cannot tolerate long trips when the pain is severe and there is only one spine surgeon in a small town. In these cases, a second surgical opinion may be waived. A second surgical opinion can sometimes be a burden to the patient. It is sometimes a waste of time and money. There is also a risk of further neurological deficits from nerve damage for delaying surgery and activities involved in the trip. A second surgical opinion is not always necessary. Sometimes, getting a second surgical opinion takes several weeks. Time is precious when a nerve is being pinched and the potential risk of permanent nerve damage exists. If the treating surgeon is professional, honest, and has a long-standing good reputation, the patient, the insurance company, or any other party might waive the need for a second surgical opinion.

Historically, insurance companies started requesting second surgical opinions to decrease the number of unnecessary operations and to reduce costs. Most recently, some insurance companies are becoming more aware that, in general, there are more honest physicians, and the need for a second surgical opinion may actually carry higher costs, not to mention the liability involved for delaying the patient's treatment. Some insurance companies have medical directors who review the medical data and make decisions for surgery. Each insurance company has its own policies.

One has to consider that a second surgical opinion could sometimes cause more confusion. Another surgeon may have his or her own methodology and rules for surgery. A surgeon can be too aggressive or too conservative. I consider each patient on an individual basis when I recommend any treatment including surgery.

A second surgical opinion can be in order when:

- The primary surgeon is rushing surgery even though the patient is getting better.
- The reputation of the surgeon is that of an aggressive physician.
- The surgeon is known to be too conservative.
- The insurance company is requesting one as an insurance policy for surgery.
- The patient wants it.

- The primary surgeon suggests getting one.

- Attorneys request it.

The patient is not only getting worse after a period of conservative treatment (four to six weeks), but the pain is well correlated with the clinical and radiological findings. Avoiding surgery may carry a great risk of nerve damage.

Pain, per se, does not necessarily warrant an emergency or urgent surgery. Patients might have low back and leg pain for several weeks, but the pain may be related to other conditions such as sacroiliac dysfunction, facet joint syndrome, hip bursitis, and other conditions mimicking sciatica. In these instances, surgery is not recommended. There are times when two conditions overlap, such as degenerative disc disease and/or a bulging disc on an MRI scan and facet joint syndrome on the same patient. One must be very careful when getting a medical history. The physical exam should be performed carefully and thoroughly.

The medical history and the exam are the pillars and foundation for diagnosis and treatment. Radiological studies assist in making a diagnosis that correlates and makes sense with the symptoms. I have seen several patients who had surgery when their pain was actually related to hip pathology, sacroiliac joint, or from the joints in the lower back. (See my list of conditions related to LBP).

Does my lower back condition put me in a different situation at work with and without surgery? Depending on the kind of work the patient was performing at the time of the injury, the patient may or may not have to change jobs or may need to have work modifications. Surgery may change work status. Surgery should increase the chances of getting back to work. But having a history of back surgery may sometimes make employers skeptical and avoid hiring these persons. It is possible for a person who had back surgery to find a job in which strenuous work is not required.

What is an IME? IME or independent medical evaluation is an evaluation usually performed by a physician familiar with injuries and disorders related to exposure (not necessarily injuries and disorders only related to work). It is a thorough medical evaluation related to body part(s) that was (were) affected during a work-related accident or exposure. An IME usually addresses several areas, such as a medical history, physical examination, diagnosis, prognosis, causation, appropriateness of treatment, impairment rating, work status, physical limitations, recommendation for diagnosis, treatment, and comments or opinions. It is a legal document used by lawyers and insurance companies in court or mediation to address the extent of injuries that resulted from an injury or exposure for reasons of medical coverage and monetary compensation. The physician performing the IME typically does not inform the patient directly of the results of the evaluation. The physician treating the patient for the injuries should not be the same one performing the IME. Physicians take special courses and seminars to get certification for performing IMEs.

When do I need to have an IME? An IME is requested when a patient, insurance company or attorney requests it to establish in a complete manner issues that I mentioned above involving an IME. Typically, it is requested when a person has reached MMI and when there is a conflict between attorneys in establishing certain aspects of a case such as causation, apportionment, impairment, and so forth.

What is an IRE (impairment rating evaluation)? An impairment rating is a percentage of impairment of a body part, organ, or system related to an injury or exposure. Impairment is found in the AMA *Guides to the Evaluation of Permanent* Impairment. The fifth edition (latest edition) is currently available. They are guides, but it is ultimately up to the physician to determine the degree of impairment.

Patients often do not know what the numbers used in an impairment rating mean, but they will ask me, "Why did you give me such a small number?" I explain to them that I get the percentage of impairment from the AMA book. The AMA *Guides to the Evaluation of Permanent Impairment* defines impairment. Impairment is related to a change in a person's health. Permanent impairment can be interpreted as any medical condition that, in time, with or without treatment, is unlikely to change over the next twelve months and has had time to heal to its optimal state. Impairment should not be considered as permanent until the clinical findings show the medical condition has been stabilized and it is likely that it will not change in twelve months. Impairment can be temporary or permanent. It is up to the physician to determine the difference and to establish these two types of impairment. The difference between these two is frequently directly related to MMI.

The kind of evaluation a physician performs on a patient may vary. For instance, a physician can perform a preemployment evaluation. There is also an IME, a disability determination, and an impairment evaluation. A disability evaluation is directly related to the determination of a person's ability to carry out certain tasks. An impairment evaluation, by definition, is the quantification of illness or injury interfering with the health status of a person that can cause physical or mental dysfunction when carrying out a task.

One must be cautious and be aware that having impairment does not mean a person is automatically disabled for all kinds of work or for Social Security benefits. A person could be impaired but not disabled, but a disabled person will most likely also be impaired. Disability involves the performance of activities of daily living (ADLs).

An impairment rating is usually performed to establish functional limitations and not disabilities. Impairment may decrease the person's ability to perform certain ADLs other than work. Disability is the incapacity of an individual to function or comply with personal, social, or occupational needs. Disability is also the incapacity to comply with rules and regulations due to severe impairment. This definition is a general one, but each state and institution may have some variations in the definition of disability. Certain factors are considered when determining disability, such as individual's skills, education, age, adaptability, work history and environmental requirements, and reasonable working modifications.

What are ADLs? Activities of daily living are usually recognized as:

- **Self-care and Personal Hygiene:** Urinating, defecation, dressing oneself, eating, brushing teeth, combing hair, bathing, and so forth
- **Sensory Function:** Hearing, seeing, smelling, tactile feeling, and tasting
- **Physical Activity:** Standing, walking, sitting, climbing stairs, and reclining
- **Travel:** Riding, driving, and flying
- **Sexual Function:** Orgasm, ejaculation, erection, and lubrication
- **Communication:** Writing, typing, seeing, speaking, and hearing
- **Nonspecialized Hand Activities:** Tactile discrimination, grasping, and lifting

ADLs do not include work tasks. Independent contractors, insurance companies, attorneys, employers, and so forth may order disability evaluations, impairment evaluations, IME, and other medical evaluations. Social Security frequently requires disability evaluations for determination of benefits. Social Security does not go hand in hand with workers' compensations insurance companies. In other words, an employee may qualify for workers' compensations benefits, but not for Social Security benefits. People tend to confuse all of these different terms. A patient who sustained an injury will not necessarily qualify for Social Security disability.

The Americans With Disabilities Act (ADA) defines disability as a "physical or mental condition that substantially limits the person's ability to one or more of the major life activities such as taking care of one's self, performing manual tasks, hearing, breathing, speaking, working, seeing, learning, and walking." Sexual intercourse may also be part of major life function. I will not delve into this other area of disability because it is related to people with disabilities in relation to equal opportunity employment. However, ADA can be applied for patients who sustained a work-related injury. I suggest reading appropriate literature related to this topic for more information.

What is an FCE or FCA (Functional Capacity Evaluation or Functional Capacity Assessment)? A Functional Capacity Evaluation or Functional Capacity Assessment is a special physical tolerance test usually performed by a certified physical therapist who is familiar with the workers' compensation setting and requests. The patient is tested physically to see how much he or she can do and what he or she cannot do. Then, the person is placed in a certain work category that may go from complete disability for any kind of physical or mental activity to partial disability.

Who requests an FCE?

- The patient
- The insurance company
- The treating physician(s)
- An attorney

What does a disability form involve? Commercial disability insurance (not workers' compensation) companies usually have a form that is sent to the treating physician(s) to be filled approximately every month or periodically until the patient is released from medical care. The physician establishes physical limitations and return to work date or estimated return to work date.

Each disability form is different, but similar questions are asked, such as:

- Diagnosis (ICD-9 and CPT)
- Has the patient ever had the same or a similar medical condition?
- Treating physician(s) information, such as name, address, medical specialty, and so forth
- Date injury or disease started
- Treatment rendered (medical or surgical) and dates of surgery
- Referring physician
- If operation, give hospital name and address and hospital stay (dates)
- Type of surgery (if any)
- Rehabilitation
- Referral to other health care providers (other physicians, physical therapists) names and addresses
- Expected disability (partial or total)

- Expected return to work (part-time or full-time and full duty or light work)
- Physical limitations (describe)
- Prognosis
- Is this a permanent or temporary medical condition and disability? Explain.
- Will the patient require further medical care, physical therapy, and so forth?

In the workers' compensation system, who sets compensation? How much compensation is provided when a person sustains a work-related injury? Insurance companies do. However, in some occasions, when a case goes to trial, a judge will set several parameters including compensation and amounts. We assist attorneys and insurance companies in providing an impairment rating on the patient for injuries or diseases sustained in the course of work. Workers' compensation insurance companies have a formula that combines other data, such as years of work, years of formal education, state rules and regulations, and so forth. Insurance companies ultimately provide disability benefits if they estimate the claim is legitimate and based on information gathered during their investigation.

Who decides when a person qualifies for disability and Social Security benefits? Patients tend to believe that we, the evaluating physicians, make these decisions. The Social Security Administration (and sometimes a judge) make these determinations.

I only provide institutions with copies of medical records (if I have treated the patient), but it is to the discretion of the government agency or institution to approve disability and benefits. It is true, however, the physician's medical records play a significant role in the disability decision.

Sometimes, before disability is set, insurance companies require another medical opinion, or a formal IME. Sometimes, to establish medical disability, a court appearance is required, and an attorney is hired. Depositions with several health care providers also take place.

Workers' compensation has a special standard state form. In this form, they consistently address the same issues, such as date of injury, whether the cause of disability is sickness or injury, MMI, physical limitations (work status), impairment rating, date of release to work (full-time, part-time, with or without restrictions), and comments and remarks about the case.

What physical limitations will I have? Are they permanent or temporary? Will I be able to work? Will I be disabled permanently or temporarily? In my opinion, a patient who had lumbar disc surgery should be permanently disabled from heavy work. However, some surgeons send their patients back to full duty, heavy work after a fusion spinal surgery. This can be controversial for some physicians. Some states have their rules and work status classification. In some states, no disability is given to a patient who has low back problems, with or without surgery.

I especially recommend my postsurgical patients avoid lifting. I arbitrarily recommend a weight limitation of thirty-five pounds, but this is also relative because even lifting thirty-five pounds in an awkward position can lead to spinal injuries. Conversely, someone may lift up to fifty pounds or more. But, if following body mechanics and the appropriate ergonomics, one should be safe. At the same time, there are differences in the lifting capacity depending on the gender, physical structure, shape, fitness, and complexion.

I definitely recommend avoiding twisting and bending the lower back when a patient has had back surgery or if there is a back injury that can be exacerbated or aggravated with these activities. There is literature that states these body functions do not contribute to complications after spine surgery. In my opinion, there is a correlation between certain activities and complications. Vibration, bumpy vehicles rides, prolonged sitting and standing, bending, lifting, and stooping are some of the activities I recommend patients should after a back injury in which there has been structural damage.

Why do some patients improve with back surgery and others do not? Will I need another surgery later in life? One must consider there is no perfect surgery for the lower back. One, as a surgeon, must choose the surgery that most likely will benefit his or her patient. This is sometimes a hard decision because there is a gray area in which more than one surgical technique can be used for a particular patient. (This is when the surgeon's experience is invaluable.)

There are times when we are not one hundred percent certain of the origin of pain, or, simply and more frequently, there is more than one cause of LBP.

Often patients expect a "magic" cure or one hundred percent relief of the pain. The goals of surgery are release pressure from nerves, alleviate symptoms, and stabilize the spine if there is instability. Surgery is also indicated to avoid neurological deficits. Surgery is designed to help the patients by opening the spaces in the spine that are getting too small and narrow. There are patients who expect to cure their underlying joint and bone disease with low back surgery. Surgery on patients with underlying joint disease such as rheumatoid arthritis may aggravate the pain. One must be cautious when doing surgery and discussing the goals of surgery with the patient. Realistic expectations have to be clearly discussed.

Sometimes, surgery on patients with RA and other progressive joint and bone disease is necessary. Due to the nature of the disease, patients develop dislocations of the spine that may be dangerous, and stabilizing surgery is needed. Sometimes, these patients develop stenosis (narrowing) of the spine, and surgery is also strongly recommended. But surgery does not stop the progression of the disease.

Whereas some patients benefit significantly from surgery; others do not. One, as a surgeon, must be honest and do only what we consider necessary. Although surgeons are honest most of the time when recommending surgery, several factors may influence the surgeon when deciding a specific operation on a patient.

Who does the paperwork? Again, it is expected (by primary care physicians and insurance companies) the surgeon who performed the operation should do of all the paperwork. A physician with sound medical knowledge and understanding of the anatomy of the spine should also be able to give recommendations for physical limitations and capabilities and for periods of disability. Occupational medicine physicians should be able to help the patient with these requests. After the surgeon has discharged the patient, the primary care physician, with information obtained form the surgeon, the occupational medicine specialist, or the pain specialist, should be able to continue to assist the patient with these requests (disability forms). Sometimes, there is a small fee for filling out the forms. Workers' compensation usually has special forms that only a physician familiar with them should complete. Sometimes, there is need for special reports. The surgeon, if not familiar with these reports, may send the patient to a physician trained in disability evaluations.

These are some of the most frequent questions patients have when I see them in my office. There is always the confusion and sometimes even hard feelings between physicians because "he or she does not want to do his or her job." Primary care physicians are overwhelmed with work, or they are simply unfamiliar with disability forms and other requests from insurance companies. Surgeons get busy in the operating room for hours, and it may take from days to weeks to do the paperwork. There should be some kind of understanding between physicians, and they should work a reasonable plan to handle these situations.

There are physicians that specialize in disability evaluation, impairment rating, independent medical evaluation, and so forth. The patient can be referred to one of these physicians for assistance with these issues. Patients may be satisfied with the outcome of surgery, but, if paperwork and forms remain unfilled, an unpleasant feeling might grow between the patient, the primary care physician, and the surgeon.

I recommend consulting appropriate sources of information (AMA *Guides to the Evaluation of Permanent Impairment*) for a more complete explanation and definition of terms discussed previously, such as MMI, IME, impairment, disability, and others.

The Future of Medicine: Possible Future Treatments for LBP Patients

New spinal surgical techniques will be developed in the future. There are two different issues related to the future of medicine: one is the economical implication and the other is the diagnostic and treatment advancement.

Instead of mystically predicting the future, we have to analyze our current surgical techniques, treatments, and resources. Medical techniques will emerge in the surgery of the spine with more refinement. Disc surgery will be more a body-like material replacement procedure. There may be a time when surgery will be obsolete. It is ironic that, with our current technology (computer systems) and knowledge in physics and medicine, no stronger efforts are made to evolve more rapidly in medicine. Regenerations, genetic manipulation, sophistication of technology in the field of electronics, computing, and programming will be the future of medicine. The ability to merge technology with human body parts and organ functions could be applied for the treatment of patients with medical conditions.

Another area of advancement in the treatment of patients could be research in genetics such as gene engineering (gene manipulation for the correction of diseases). Gene models can be pictures and worked up more rapidly with our current computing systems. The creation of models will lead to the correction of diseases. The production of a regenerating gene will reproduce disc tissue again. The key to curing many ailments and to longevity lies in the world of genetics and its application in key body organs and glands such as the pineal gland and hypothalamus.

Other more technical futuristic advances may be related to the use of transcutaneous or percutaneous healing techniques with the use of computing and programming systems that apply certain known forces such as radiation, laser, heat, cold, or unknown forces yet to be discovered. Forces that can be applied through the intact skin. Incisions, sutures, blood loss, and all the trauma associated with open surgery will be part of rudimentary medicine. One of the most recent advances in surgery of the spine is the replacement of a disc in lumbar and cervical surgery (artificial disc). This technique has been practiced in Europe for some time.

In time, there will be no need for even any needles, surgery, or painful procedures. There may be all "closed" medical techniques for diagnosis and treatment. As we speak, there is a gamma knife or radiosurgery treatment for certain tumors. This is only the tip of the iceberg that could lead toward more sophisticated techniques that apply energy to certain deep body part for the treatment of certain ailments.

Future of Neuroradiology. New MRI machines and radiodiagnostic studies will be available someday, and machines will give a more realistic view of the body. The current MRI scan machine provides a picture of a body part while lying down. We still do not have an MRI scan that will do a test while standing to see the true anatomy, physiology, and mechanics of the spine. (There is recent research about it.) New generations of MRI scan machine are currently being used in which an intraoperative picture can be obtained. These machines are extremely expensive because, not only the machine will have to be adapted for the operating room, but the operative instruments would also have to be MRI-compatible (titanium). These adaptations in the operating room would be exorbitantly expensive. New neurodiagnostic machines will come to the market in which other kinds of energy and biological fields and body components will be used to make a neurobiological and neurophysiological diagnosis rather than only an anatomical, mechanical picture given for diagnosis. Someday, there will be a machine able to combine anatomical and physiological information at the same time (such as MRI-PET integrated) that will yield both anatomical and physiological information of a body part or organ in a more realistic and efficient manner.

The Economical Future of Medicine. It seems to me that medical resources will progressively be more restricted as the global economy staggers. Consumerism will have to change to new techniques for recycling. Many countries have already experienced this situation with economical restrictions and on the use of resources in a more practical way for the medical field. In the future, medicine in this country may become socialized or semisocialized. In socialized medicine, people do not have the choice of selecting a determined physician. The decisions patients make will be more restricted in the future. The health care reform was created primarily to shift economical resources of the national budget into other areas of more importance for the government.

Socialized medicine is a system that has been practiced by several countries in the world. Physicians in some countries do not have sophisticated technology to treat people. The tort reform, particularly, malpractice capitation will be a must to avoid further inflation of the economy in general. It is estimated the government loses about $28 billion a year from the direct cost of liability insurance and the indirect cost of defensive medicine.

The Last Words but Not the Least

- I do not recommend using this books as a source of medical information for legal issues because there are appropriate medical textbooks with scientific accurate information that is required for such cases.

- Treatment may vary as patients present with different conditions and with different set of personal, social, and constitutional situations. I do not demote or criticize any institution or particular practitioner of the art of healing.
- I recommend consulting with your primary care physicians and spine surgeon for advice for the treatment of LBP.
- Do not be distrustful of the medical establishment.
- Use common sense when being treated, and never assume facts. Ask questions!
- Be cautious when checking the media and other sources of information when seeking advice for treatment.
- Always tell your physicians all of your medical conditions, recent infections, allergies, medications, and remedies you are taking. Bring a list of medications to the hospital or clinic if consulting a physician or having surgery. Repeat the same information to your nurses if you are having back surgery.
- Comply with your physician's recommendations.
- Gene therapy is still experimental, but, in my opinion, it is the future of the treatment for LBP and other disorders.
- Notice I have mentioned medical and clinical entities and new diagnosis that still have not been published in regular textbooks or journals. These new conditions are:
  - The "lateral recess syndrome with a taut ligamentum flavum" in which there is a tense ligamentum flavum that abnormally traps the nerve root underneath the facet joint and a shortened pedicle. This condition tends to occur in relatively young patients. This syndrome is sometimes associated with congenital shortened pedicles. Patients typically have radicular pain (leg pain) with unremarkable radiological studies but with a positive EMG/NCV and SSEP studies. Note that shorten pedicle in the spine have already been described in medical textbooks, but the observation of the association of a "taut" ligament has not been described.
  - There is also the "engorge nerve root vein syndrome" clinical entity characterized by large dilated veins that wrap the nerve root.

    These conditions can also cause leg pain, and the typical radiological studies are unremarkable, again with positive SSEP and EMG/NCV. Vascular malformations, however, are well-known medical entities already known by spine surgeons. The "engorged nerve root vein" has not clearly been studied. This phenomenon may be related to chronic nerve irritation and inflammatory reaction with neovascular formation. Recent articles have described this medical entity.

- I have also observed an entity that is relatively common—conjoined nerve root or duplicated nerve root. This condition may present on one side or on both sides (right and left). The nerves might be separate, or they may run into one single nerve sheath (enlarged nerve root). One must be aware of nerve root tumors and other known entities.

- This book contains some modifications to the traditional low back exercises that primary care physicians and other spine surgeons have routinely recommended to their patients. They are personal observations.

- In this book, I have described a new syndrome (NONRAS), Non-Osteoarthritis and Non-Rheumatoid Arthritis Syndrome.

- There are variations on the physical exam:
  - "The one-foot tiptoe test" is a test I designed to test muscle strength, particularly in the lower legs.
  - The "squatting on one leg"
  - The straight-leg-raising (SLR) usually elicits LBP with radiation into the leg(s) when there is a "pinched nerve." The SLR and extension of the foot while the patient lies down on his or her back may cause more LBP and leg pain. It is only another way of performing the SLR. The SLR test is positive not only on patients with a disc herniation.
  - When the physician gently taps the patient's foot (bottom) with the fist while the patient lies down on an exam table on his or her back, LBP and leg pain may increase on a patient with suspected disc herniation in the lumbar spine. But again, this sign is not specific and not sensitive.

These are some of my clinical observations. Some have already been described, but I have added variations on the exam to detect a patient with a "pinched nerve." During private practice, it is difficult to publish new discoveries in medicine.

It should be understood that back surgery is not the "magic bullet." I do not promote back surgery in all patients with LBP. Most patients with LBP do not need surgery. Conservative and semiconservative treatments are generally more beneficial than surgery in most cases of LBP. However, I disagree that only ten percent of patients with a slipped disc require surgery. I would recommend analyzing and studying patients on a case-by-case basis. I also disagree that only a low percentage of patients improve with surgery as stated in some textbooks and other literature.

I think there are many patients that, for fear of surgery or due to misinformation, suffer with LBP for several months and years. This is unfair. I also have experienced in my practice that patients do not fare well when surgery was postponed when they were waiting to improve with "conservative treatment." I do not speak as a surgeon. I speak as a physician, and the job of a surgeon is the opposite of what people and colleagues think. It is not to operate on all patients we see in the office. Instead, it is to keep them away from surgery and to operate only on the ones we honestly think will improve.

All patients who suffer from LBP, regardless of their social, financial, racial, or cultural status will learn some important information by reading this book.

There are medical conditions that just do not have a cure. However, one, as a physician, can alleviate pain and suffering. The art of medicine resides in letting Mother Nature take its course. The key to practicing medicine is not to interfere with Mother Nature and to avoid further damage with our treatments.

Mario A. Gutierrez, M.D.

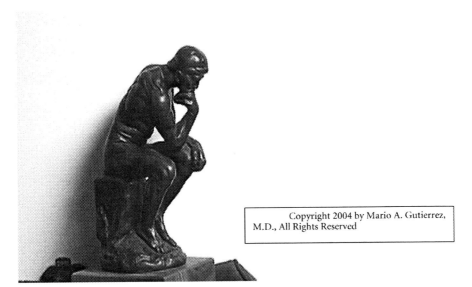

"There is still a long journey into the fathoms of the human body."
Mario A. Gutierrez, M.D.

MEDICAL ABBREVIATIONS

These are abbreviations of professional associations and titles that may relate to the treatment of patients with LBP:

ABA American Board of Anesthesia

AAN American Academy of Neurology

AANS American Association of Neurological Surgeons

AAOS American Academy of Orthopaedic Surgeons

APMA Anesthesiology and Pain Management Association

AAPM American Academy of Pain Management (Medicine)

ABIME American Board of Independent Medical Examiners

AMA American Medical Association

BM Bachelor of Medicine

BSN Bachelor of Science in Nursing

CA Certified Acupuncturist

CAMT Certified Acupressure Massage Therapist

CMT Certified Massage Therapist

DC Doctor of Chiropractic

DHANP Doctor of Homeopathic Academy of Naturopathic Physicians

D.Hom. (Med) Diplomat of Homeopathic Medicine

Dipl. Ac. Diplomat of Acupuncture

Dipl. CH. Diplomat of Chinese Herbs

DO Doctor of Osteopathy

DOM Doctor of Oriental Medicine (or OMD)

D.Sc. Doctor of Science

FAAFP Fellow of the American Academy of Family Practice

FAAPM Fellow of the American Academy of Physical Medicine

F.Ac.A. Fellow of the Acupuncture Association

FACS Fellow of the American College of Surgeons

FIACA Fellow of the International Academy of Certified Acupuncturists

FICC Fellow of the International College of Chiropractors

FICS Fellow of the International College of Surgeons

FNAAOM Fellow of the National Academy of Acupuncture and Oriental Medicine

FNTOS Fellow of the Natural Therapeutic and Osteopathic Society

HMD Homeopathic Medical Doctor

L.Ac. License Acupuncturist
LMT License Massage Therapist
CMA Certified Medical Assistant
CNP Certified Nurse Practitioner
CPA Certified Physician Assistant
CNA Certified Nurses Aide
EOHSI Environmental and Occupational Health Science Institute
EOM Environmental and Occupational Medicine
M.Ac.OM Master of Acupuncture and Oriental Medicine
MD Medical Doctor
MDC Master Doctor of Chiropractor
MPH Master of Public Health
MS Master of Science
NCCA National Commission of the Certification of Acupuncturist
ND Doctor of Naturopathy
NMD Neuropathic Medical Doctor
OHIM Occupational Health and Industrial Medicine
Occ Med Occupational Medicine
OMM Osteopath Manipulative Medicine
PM&R Physical Medicine and Rehabilitation
RN Registered Nurse
RPT Register Physical Therapist
Other Abbreviations and Medical Terms
Some most commonly used medical terms and abbreviations:
ACJ acromioclavicular joint
AP or PA anteroposterior or posterior anterior (as for X-rays)
ACL anterior crucial ligament (knee)
ADLs activities of daily living
Blue Code means a patient is in cardiorespiratory arrest and requires immediate attention and CPR
CA cancer
CNS central nervous system
CTS carpal tunnel syndrome
CFS chronic fatigue syndrome
C/O complains of...
DNR do not resuscitate
DDD degenerative disc disease
DJD degenerative joint disease
DVT deep venous thrombosis
FM fibromyalgia

FX fracture
GSW gunshot wound
H/A headache; high anxiety; hemolytic anemia.
H/O history of…
HNP herniated nucleus pulposus
HTN hypertension
IV intravenous (IVF: IV fluids)
IBS irritable bowel syndrome
Lac. laceration
LBP low back pain
LE lower extremities (RLE and LLE; right and left)
LED lupus erythematosus disseminatus
LP lumbar puncture
METS metastasis (spread of cancer to one more or multiple organs). Sometimes, these are organs away from the original cancerous organ (e.g., lung cancer and brain metastasis).
MI myocardiac infarction (heart attack)
MS multiple sclerosis
MVA motor vehicle accident (MCA: motorcycle accident)
N/V nausea and vomiting
PE pulmonary embolism
ROM range of motion
RA rheumatoid arthritis
RLS Restless Leg Syndrome
SIJ sacroiliac joint
SLR straight-leg-raising (Lasègue's sign)
STAT sudden turn around time (that is, a medical emergency requires immediate medical attentions and/or X-rays or labs)
SX surgery
TMJ temporomandibular joint
UE upper extremities (RUP and LUE)
UTI urinary tract infection
VS vital signs (BP: blood pressure) (RR: respiratory rate) (HR: heart rate or pulse) (T: temperature) (U/O: urinary output) (I+O: in and out fluids)
Lab Abbreviations
BMP basic metabolic panel or blood chemistry (CMP: comprehensive metabolic panel)
CBC complete blood count
CT scan computerized tomography
CXR chest X-ray

CSF cerebrospinal fluid
EEG electroencephalogram
EMG/NCV electromyography and nerve conduction velocity
ETOH alcohol
EKG or ECG electrocardiogram
LFT liver function test
MRI magnetic resonance imaging
MRA magnetic resonance angiography
PFT pulmonary function test
SSEP Somatosensory Evoked Potentials (Motor and Sensory)
U/A urinalysis (C+S: culture and sensitivity)
More abbreviations (frequently used by workers' compensation)
W/C workers' compensation
IME independent medical evaluation
IR impairment rating
MMI maximum medical improvement

MEDICAL ORDERS

Several years ago, medical orders in Europe were traditionally written in Latin. To date, these words are still used:

A.C. ante cibum (before meals)
ADL activities of daily living
AMA against medical advice
BID twice a day (medication) (bis in die)
BR bed rest
c and s with or without (also s and s)
D/C discharge
DX diagnosis
HOB head of the bed
HS at bedtime (hora somni)
IV intravenous (IM: intramuscular) (SQ: subcutaneous)
NPO or (NPO/HS) nothing by mouth at bedtime (*nulla per os hora somni*).
NBM nothing by mouth
OD once daily
OM every morning (omni mane)
ON every night (omni nocte) (QN: every night) (QM: every morning)
OTC over-the-counter
PC post meals (post cibum)
Per os by mouth
PO postoperative (PO or by mouth)
PMN past midnight
PRN as the occasion arises; as needed. (pro re nata)
PR per rectum
PDR Physician's Desk Reference
QHS every day at bedtime
QD every day (quaque die)
QH every hour (quaque hora) (Q1H, Q2H, Q3H, and so forth: every hour, two hours, three hours, and so forth)
QID four times per day (quarter in die)
QOD every other day
QOH every other hour
R/O rule out

RX prescription
Susp suspension
Syr syrup
TID three times a day (medication) (ter in die)
TSP teaspoonful
Tab tablet (pill)

MEDICAL GLOSSARY

Absorb: to assimilate

Adenopathy: enlargement of lymph glands (usually)

Afebrile: without fever

Algorithm: a step-by-step process of solving a problem; a way of following certain procedures in an organized manner; flowchart; protocol.

Allograft: a graft of the same animal species but different genotype

Ambulation: walking

Analgesic: pain reliever or painkiller

Aneurysm: a dilatation or sac on the wall of a blood vessel (usually an artery). An aneurysm has a thick wall and can rupture and cause profuse bleeding.

Angioma: a tumor made of blood vessels. It is typically benign but highly hemorrhagic when trying to remove.

Angioedema: swelling or edema caused by dilatation of blood vessels and increased permeability manifesting as large wheels (under the skin)

Ankylosis: stiffness or immobility of a joint (fusion of a joint) related to disease or surgery

Anoxia: lack of oxygen supply into the tissues despite adequate blood perfusion

Antalgic: posture or activity adopted to avoid pain (for example, limping is an antalgic gait)

Anterior: toward the front or situated at the front

Anticoagulants: medication used to avoid coagulation of blood. Anticoagulants make an individual bleed excessively.

Arachnoid: thin membrane between the inner part of the dura and the outer layer of the brain or spinal cord (pia). They constitute the meninges. When cerebrospinal fluid (CSF) accumulates between layers of meninges, they can form an arachnoid cyst.

Articulation (articular): joint

Asepsis: without infection

Asymmetry: unequal size or form when comparing right and left side of the body; opposite of symmetry

Atelectasis: collapsing of the alveoli (lung). The alveoli are the small saclike endings of the bronchioles, and they are full of air. Collapsing of the alveoli can cause fluid accumulation and pneumonia. This is one of the most frequent causes of fever after surgery or patients have been bedridden.

Atrophy: decrease in size of a cell, organ, tissue, or body part related to wasting away of cells

Autoimmune: immunologic reaction of the body to its own body tissues

Autologous or **autograft:** a graft of the same individual (as in bone graft taken out of the fibula bone or the iliac bone of the patient undergoing surgery for a spinal fusion)

Avascular: without blood vessels or blood supply. Tissues usually die without blood supply.

Axial: a line through the center of a body in a horizontal plane, usually referring to horizontal cuts or slices a structure or the body. (Sagittal cuts are vertical slices of a structure or body.)

Axilla: armpit. It is the inner or most medial part of a shoulder and is lateral to the body. When referring to nerves, it is the inner part of the nerve.

Baseline: a value obtained as a reference point for further comparisons

Benign: nonmalignant. (Benign tumors do not typically spread in the body or distant organs as in cancer.)

Biofeedback: voluntary control of vital signs and other body functions using certain techniques of self-control and learning techniques

Biomechanics: the use of mechanical forces to living organisms

Biopsy: the removal of tissue for microscopic analysis for diagnosis

Bursa: a sac made of tissue around the joints. There is usually fluid that reduces friction between tendons, ligaments, and bone. Inflammation of these saclike structures is called bursitis, and it can be rather painful. Accumulation of fluid in the bursa can become a cyst (synovial cyst).

Cadaver: corpse; dead body

Calcification: deposit of calcium in tissue (usually in soft tissues)

Canal: a small or narrow channel or passage (spinal canal)

Capsule: a structure enclosed by tissue and sometimes holds fluid (as in joints)

Carcinosis: carcinoma (related to cancer)

Cardiologist: a physician specializing in heart conditions

Cartilage: tissue usually located between joints. It can be fibrous, elastic, and hyaline. Fibrocartilage (intervertebral disc) is made of fibrous tissue and some content of calcium (making it look like crabmeat).

Catheter: a tube use to place in body parts to drain fluid. It is usually a plastic tube that comes in different sizes.

Cauda Equina: a cluster of spinal nerves descending from the spinal cord below the end of the spinal cord (conus) in the spinal canal

Caudal: inferior or bottom of a body

Causalgia: a burning pain associated with nerve damage (usually sharp nerve injuries)

Cellulitis: inflammatory reaction of the soft tissues that is usually associated with infectious processes

Cephalic: the upper end of the body (toward the head)

Claudication: leg pain usually associated when walking and with improvement when resting. Claudication can be vascular (ischemia) or neurogenic (compression of the spinal nerves).

Claustrophobia: afraid of being in close and narrow spaces

Clinical: *klinikos* (bed)

Coagulopathy: state of difficulty coagulating blood, possibly related to disorders, poisons, and medications

Concomitant: occurring at the same time (for example, two diseases or disorders happening at the same time)

Coccygodynia: pain localized to the coccyx (due to trauma or disease)

Congenital: present at the time of birth

Connective (tissue): lax tissue in the body that connects other tissues and organs

Contracture: shortening of muscle tissue, making a limb be stiff in one position and usually keeping a joint in flexion or bending position

Contrast: (in medicine) a reference to the use of dyes that are usually non-toxic and tolerated by the body. In large amounts, it can be toxic (kidney, liver, and so forth).

Decompression: a procedure in medicine (usually) used to relieve pressure in which structures, organs, or canals are opened

Deficit: deficiency or lack of

Degenerate: to change from a higher or normal form to a less quality or deteriorated form (degenerative condition)

Dermatome: a strip of skin innervated by a spinal nerve

Disc or Disk: a reference (usually) to the intervertebral disc in the spine. Cushing oval fibrocartilage structure with jelly-like soft material in the inner or center part of the disc (nucleus) maintained or held in place by the annulus or fibrous tissue (ligament).

Discogenic: pain related to the disc (usually back pain and/or leg pain)

Diskitis: inflammation of the disc usually related to infection or arthritis

Dysesthesia: abnormal skin feeling, such as burning, numbness, tingling, and so forth. Unpleasant abnormal sensation triggered by normal stimuli. Paresthesia is usually heightened sensitivity also felt as numbness, tingling, or prickling.

Dysfunction: malfunction. Impairment or disturbances in function.

Dyskinesia: a defect to perform voluntary movement

Dyspareunia: painful intercourse

Dysraphism: a failure to fuse bone or organs (skin, spine, brain, spinal cord, and so forth) in the fetal or embryogenic stage. (Spinal dysraphia or dysrhaphism is the lack of fusion of normal bones such as vertebrae.)

Dystonia: It is related to prolonged muscle contraction and sometimes causes twitching, repetitive movements, or abnormal and fixed postures.

Dystrophy: a lack of nutrition that causes certain disorders. (In muscular dystrophy, there is lack of nutrients to the muscle, which causes it to waste away.) Dystrophy is usually hereditary or genetic-related.

Dura Mater: the outermost, thickest layer of the meninges (membrane or cover of the brain and spinal cord)

Dysrhythmia: abnormal rhythm (brain waves, heart, and so forth)

Eccentric: away from the center

Edema: swelling; fluid accumulation in the soft tissues.

Embolism: a sudden clogging or blocking of an artery (by a blood clot or foreign body)

Empirical: practice based on experience rather than on scientific information

Endocrine: related to internal secretion usually of hormones (by glands such as the pituitary, thyroid, and so forth)

Endorphin: a substance related to morphine that is produced by the body to raise pain threshold

Endoscopy: an examination of usually small areas with an endoscope, a usually tubular instrument with a light source that is sometimes attached to a camera and a monitor for visualization of internal body organs and parts

Enzyme: a protein produced by a cell to increase catalysis in biochemical reactions of a cell

Epidemiology: the study of frequency, distribution, and relations of several aspects of a disease in a community

Ergonomics: the science of the interrelation of the human and work and the factors affecting the efficient use of the body

Etiology: the study of the causes of a disease. It is also used to refer to the cause of a disease (for example, the *etiology* of pneumonia can be viral).

Excision: removing by means of cutting

Extravasation: discharge or escape of blood or other fluid from a contained place, blood vessel, or organ

Extrusion: something out of place (displaced) and out of its normal position

Extubation: the act of removing an endotracheal tube

Exudate: fluid accumulation inside a body cavity, usually because of inflammation and infection (not always). Transudate is also accumulation of fluid, but there is less protein, cells, and solid components than in an exudate.

Facet: a smooth or small, hard surface (in a bone) that is usually in contact with another bone and becomes a joint

Fluoroscope: a radiological devices used to visualize (in a monitor) internal structures or bones by means of X-ray shadows

Foramen: a passage or hole usually in bones (for blood vessels, nerves, and other structures)

Forceps: a surgical instrument with a handle (usually double–bladed) for grasping tissue

Fusion: the act of merging or uniting two or more objects

Ganglion: a group of nerve cell bodies usually located outside the central nervous system (with some exceptions)

Hematoma: a blood clot (extravasated blood) usually localized in an organ, space, or body tissue

Hernia: a protrusion of part of an organ or tissue through an abnormal opening

Holistic (Medicine): the comprehensive care of a patient (physical, emotional, spiritual, and economical)

Hormone: a chemical substance or protein produced by cells that affects the function of target organs and has a regulatory effect on cells

Hydrocephalus: accumulation of excessive spinal fluid in the cerebral or brain ventricles (normal spaces inside the brain)

Hypoxia: decreased oxygen supply in the tissues despite adequate blood flow

Iatrogenic: adverse outcome because of treatment or surgery (caused by a health care provider)

Idiopathic: of unknown cause (for example, a disease or syndrome)

Immunity: a reference (usually) to the body's own self-defense against noxious stimuli, tumor, or infection disorders. It involves the body's self-defense biological system.

Incidence: the number of new cases of a particular disease observed in a certain period of time. It is the rate at which certain conditions occur in a determined population and in a certain time.

Infarct: area of ischemia or lack of blood supply due to occlusion of a blood vessel with subsequent damage to tissues and organs

Infiltrate: the act of passing into or through a substance or a space

Internist: a physician specializing in the study of internal organs (and disorders)

Intraoperative: activities that occur during surgery

Intubation: the act of applying an endotracheal tube

Ischemia: decreased or lack of blood supply to an organ than can lead to necrosis and damage

Kyphosis: increased curve of the spine (increased convexity) when seen from the side

Lesion: any discontinuity of tissue (tumor or any mass) or loss of function of a body part that can be caused by trauma or disease

Ligament: bands of connective tissue that bind together the articular ends of bones (joints)

Lipoma: a fatty tumor that usually is benign

Lordosis: an increased forward curve of the spine when seen from the side

Lumbago: LBP (any cause)

Lymphatic: special system carrying body fluid, blood vessel-like system

Lymphedema: swelling due to accumulation of fluid due to blockage of the lymphatic system

Macrophage: large defense cells part of the immune system of the body

Malignant: related to cancer

Medial: pertaining to a location in the middle or center of a structure. Referring towards the midline.

Meninges: pertaining to the three covers of the brain and spinal cord: dura, arachnoid, and pia mater (from the outside to the inside)

Metastasis: the migration or movement of body cells or bacteria from one part of the body to another

Morbid: unhealthy state, condition, or habit that usually leads to a disease

Munchausen Syndrome: the practice of a person performing acts of selfmutilation or injury to feign illness. From Baron Karl F.H. von Munchausen, fictitious baron created by Rudolph Raspe in the eighteenth century.

Myelitis: inflammation of the spinal cord

Myelomeningocele: protrusion of hernia of the spinal cord and meninges through a bone defect in the vertebral column

Myocardium: a reference to the heart muscle. (Myocardial infarction is the lack of oxygen to the myocardium that can cause damage to the heart muscle.)

Necrosis: cell death

Neovascularization: new growth of blood vessels. (**Neoformation:** new formation, growth, neoplasm, or regeneration.)

Neoplasm: abnormal tissue formation, as in tumor (growth). A neoplasm can be benign or malignant.

Neuropathy: pertaining to any dysfunction of the nerves (usually the peripheral nerves)

Neurotransmitter: a substance released by a brain cell (neuron) for activation or inhibition of a brain function

Nucleus Pulposus: the elastic, semi-fluid material in the center of a disc

Osteoarthritis: degenerative disease of the joints that is not inflammatory in nature, better known as "arthritis."

Osteoarthropathy: a reference to any disease or disorder of the joints and bones

Osteoarthrosis: pertaining to chronic inflammatory bone disease

Osteomalacia: a reference to softening of the bones due to poor or impaired mineralization

Osteomyelitis: bone infection

Osteopenia: a decrease in the bone mass per unit of volume but not as severe as in osteoporosis

Osteophyte: commonly known as "spurs." They are represented as ridges or outgrowths on the bones (usually on the edges of the vertebral bodies and bones of the feet). They sometimes pinch nerves or the spinal cord, resulting in painful conditions.

Osteoporosis: a weakening of the bones due to severe decrease in body mass (usually calcium). The bones become brittle and translucent on X-rays.

Osteosclerosis: abnormal density and hardening of the bone

Palliative: a drug, procedure, or agent that relieves (pain) without curing a condition

Paresis: muscle weakness (**Paraplegia:** complete paralysis of the legs) (**Quadriplegia:** paralysis of the arms and legs)

Pathologic: pertaining to a disease or disorder caused by a morbid condition. Pathology is the study of the nature and cause of a disease (including the changes in the structure and function of an organ). Pathology also refers to a medical condition, disease, or disorder. Macroscopic and microscopic studies of the body and body fluids are made to determine the etiology (or cause of a disease) and determine causes of death in pathology as a science.

Percutaneous: something felt (on palpation) or performed through the skin. It usually refers to a procedure performed inside the body through a skin incision. Usually, for the performance of a percutaneous procedure, endoscopic instruments are used.

Placebo: a harmless substance (usually) given to a patient in lieu of medication. Patients may experience improvement due to psychological component of a disease.

Pneumothorax: collapsing of a lung, usually due to a puncture. (Spontaneous collapsing can occur.)

Posterior: situated at the back

Prevalence: the total number of cases of a disease in a population in a given time

Prophylactic: pertaining to avoidance (ward off) of disease by means of prevention. Avoidance of a harmful factor(s) or use of medication or vaccination to prevent disease.

Prosthesis: a device used to replace a body part

Pseudoarthrosis: failure of fusion or lack of callous formation after a bone fracture or an attempted surgical bone fusion. This condition can be painful and tends to cause instability.

Pseudomeningocele: accumulation of spinal fluid in a tissue pocket usually under the skin

Pulmonologist: a physician specializing in lung conditions

Radiculitis: inflammation of a spinal nerve usually causing pain radiating down an extremity or limb (usually related to irritation or compression of a spinal nerve)

Radiculopathy: disease of a spinal nerve that is usually associated with radicular pain (pain radiating down an extremity in the distribution of a spinal nerve)

Radionuclide: radioactive nuclide

Regional: area with more or less defined boundaries

Retrograde: anything going or traveling backwards

Retroperitoneal: pertaining to structures behind the peritoneal cavity

Rhizotomy: transection or the creation of a lesion of a nerve root, usually performed for intractable pain. (It can be performed surgically, chemically, or utilizing heat).

Rotoscoliosis: a curve of the spine sideways and rotation of the spine on its own axis

Sagittal: side view of an object

Sciatica: pain or neuralgia along the trajectory of the sciatic nerve (pain behind the hip and leg)

Scoliosis: sideway deviation of the spine and a front or back view of the spine

Seroma: accumulation of fluid under the skin made of serum or blood products and exudate, usually appearing after surgery when there has been an empty space (gap) left in the soft tissues. Seromas are usually aseptic (free of infection), but they can become infected.

Somatization: body conversion of disease due to mental or psychological states

Somatoform: symptoms related to psychological origin and resembling physical disorders

Spine bifida: defective splitting or lack of fusion of the vertebral column through which the spinal cord or meninges may or may not protrude

Spirometry: pertaining to the measurement of lung capacity and other lung functions

Spondylitis: inflammation of the vertebrae

Spondylosis: a reference (usually) to degenerative arthritis or osteoarthritis of the spine. It can be associated with pressure over the nerves, resulting in LBP and/or radicular pain.

Spondylolysis: breaking down of a vertebra. Usually, there is breakage or failure of union of vertebral parts.

Spondylolisthesis: slipping forward of one vertebra over another. (Retrolisthesis is slipping of one vertebra over another backwards.)

Sprain: some fibers of a ligament rupturing in a joint

Stenosis: narrowing of a space or canal

Steri-Strips: butterfly-like or small material (like a Band-Aid) applied to a wound to approach the edges

Strain: overexertion of a muscle ("pulled muscle")

Stroke: Strokes can be ischemic (lack of blood supply and necrosis), or they can be hemorrhagic. They usually result in neurological impairment.

Subarachnoid: the space between the arachnoid and the pia mater (filled with CSF or spinal fluid)

Subluxation: dislocation, usually referring to a joint that slips out of place

Sutures: a reference (usually) to stitches in a wound. (But, in anatomy, a suture is a joint of the skull bones.)

Sympathetic and parasympathetic: a reference to a special system in the central nervous system that controls autonomic functions, such as sweat, blood vessel constriction and dilatation, bladder and rectal function, and vital signs

Syndrome: a group of symptoms and signs in which the cause, natural history, and treatment are not usually well-known

Synovia: viscous fluid found inside joints, bursa, and tendon sheaths

Tendon: connective (fibrous) tissue that connects or attaches muscle to bones

Thrombosis: a formation of a blood clot inside a blood vessel

Tort: a reference to a wrongful act or injury from one person to another

Transcutaneous: percutaneous. Effect through the skin or structure felt under the skin. Medications and needles are applied percutaneously for injections or removal of substances. (**Transdermal:** medicine applied in a gel-like matrix to be delivered through the skin.)

The following roots or endings in a medical term mean:

"ectomy" = Removal (e.g., colectomy, gastrectomy, laminectomy, and so forth)

"otomy" = Opening and decompression (e.g., colostomy, laminotomy, gastrostomy, and so forth)

"itis" = Inflammation (e.g., appendicitis, cholecystitis, cellulites, meningitis, arachnoiditis, and so forth)

978-0-595-34117-7
0-595-34117-9

CPSIA information can be obtained at www.ICGtesting.com
Printed in the USA
LVOW05s1842220514

386947LV00001B/263/A